WORKING TOGETHER TO MANAGE DIABETES

A Guide for Pharmacy, Podiatry, Optometry, and Dental Professionals

Credits and Acknowledgements

This material was developed by the National Diabetes Education Program's Pharmacy, Podiatry, Optometry, and Dental Professionals' Work Group. NDEP would like to acknowledge the following work group members for their work on the revision:

Barbara Aung, D.P.M.

W. Lee Ball, Jr., O.D.

Joseph M. Caporusso, D.P.M.

JoAnn Gurenlian, R.D.H., Ph.D.

Stuart T. Haines, Pharm.D., F.C.C.P., F.A.S.H.P., B.C.P.S.

Mimi Hartman, M.A., R.D., C.D.E.

Cynthia Heard, O.D.

Cynthia Hodge, D.M.D.

Milissa A. Rock, R.Ph., C.D.E.

George W. Taylor, III, D.M.D., Dr.P.H.

Jaime R. Torres, D.P.M., M.S.

NDEP also thanks the following individuals for their work on the original Working Together document upon which this revision is based:

Norma Bowyer, O.D., M.P.H., F.A.A.O.

Caswell Evans, D.D.S., M.P.H.

Deborah Faucette, R.Ph.

Lawrence Harkless, D.P.M.

Tom Murray, Pharm.D.

Ross Taubman, D.P.M.

In addition, the following NDEP staff at the Centers for Disease Control and Prevention (CDC) and the National Institutes of Health (NIH) contributed to the review and revision of these materials:

Pamela Allweiss, M.D.

Sabrina Harper, M.S.

Joanne Gallivan, M.S., R.D.

Jane Kelly, M.D.

Linda Orgain, M.P.H.

Continuing Education Credit

The Centers for Disease Control and Prevention is accredited by the Accreditation Council for Continuing Medical Education (ACCME) to provide continuing medical education for physicians.

The Centers for Disease Control and Prevention designates this educational activity for a maximum of 1.25 category 1 credits toward the AMA Physician's Recognition Award. Each physician should claim only those credits that he/she actually spent in the activity.

 The Centers for Disease Control and Prevention is accredited by the Accreditation Council for Pharmacy Education as a provider of continuing pharmacy education. This program is a designated event for pharmacists to receive .1 Contact Hour in pharmacy education. The Universal Program Number is 387-603-06-042-H-01.

This activity for 1.25 contact hours is provided by the Centers for Disease Control and Prevention, which is accredited as a provider of continuing education in nursing by the American Nurses Credentialing Center's Commission on Accreditations.

The CDC has been reviewed and approved as an Authorized Provider by the International Association for Continuing Education and Training (IACET) 8405 Greensboro Drive, Suite 800, McLean, Virginia 22102. The CDC has awarded 0.1 CEUs to participants who successfully complete this program.

To receive continuing education credit for this course:

- Go to the CDC/ATSDR Training and Continuing Education Online at http://www.cdc.gov/phtnonline. If you have not registered as a participant, click on New Participant to create a user ID and password; otherwise click on "Participant Login" and log in.

- Once logged on to the CDC/ATSDR Training and Continuing Education Online Web site, you will be on the "Participant Services" page. Click on "Search and Register." Enter the course number (SS1126) or a keyword under "Keyword Search." Click on "View."

- Click on the course title (Working Together to Manage Diabetes). Select the type of CE credit you would like to receive and then "Submit." Three demographic questions will come up. Complete the questions and then "Submit." A message will come up thanking you for registering for the course. If you have already completed it, you may choose to go straight to the evaluation and posttest. Complete the evaluation and "Submit." Complete the posttest and "Submit." A record of your course completion will be located in the "Transcript and Certificate" section.

- When asked for a verification code, please use PPOD-07.
- Continuing education credits for additional professions may be offered in the future. Visit www.cdc.gov/phtnonline for updates.

If you have any questions or problems please contact: CDC/ATSDR Training and Continuing Education Online, 1-800-41TRAIN or 404-639-1292. E-mail at ce@cdc.gov.

The materials and continuing education credits are free. Requirements for obtaining continuing education include reading *Working Together to Manage Diabetes: A Guide for Pharmacists, Podiatrists, Optometrists, and Dental Professionals* and the *Working Together to Manage Diabetes* patient education poster, registering on the Centers for Disease Control and Prevention's continuing education Web site (www.cdc.gov/phtnonline), and completing an evaluation form and posttest.

Release Date: January 24, 2007

CDC, our planners, and our content experts wish to disclose that they have no financial interests or other relationships with the manufacturers of commercial products, suppliers of commercial services, or commercial supporters, with the exception of Dr. Haines, who discloses that he is a Merck minor shareholder, and Dr. Taylor, who discloses that he has received research grants from NIH/NIDCR, Blue Cross Blue Shield of Michigan, and the Foundation for Oral Health for diabetes-related research projects, and he is a scientific consultant for the Colgate Palmolive Company. Content will not include any discussion of the unlabeled use of a product or a product under investigational use.

NDEP would like to thank the following individuals who pilot tested the materials for continuing education credits:

Theresa Aldridge, O.D.
Chris Allen, R.Ph., M.P.H.
Pam Allweiss, M.D., M.P.H.
Gary Baker, R.Ph., M.B.A.
Silvia Benincaso, M.P.H., R.D., C.D.E.
Dan Bintz, O.D.
David Bordeaux, D.D.S., M.A.G.D.
Heidi Brainerd, M.S., R.Ph.
Kat Chinn, R.N., M.S.,F.N.P.
Dawn Clary, O.D.
Gay Crawford, R.D., M.P.H., C.D.E.
Eugene Dannels, D.P.M.
Michael Duenas, O.D.
Charles Edwards, D.P.M.
Kris Ernst, B.S.N., R.N., C.D.E.
Pamela Euliss, R.D.H.
Beth Finnson, R.D.H., M.P.H.
Adam Gordon, O.D., M.P.H.
Chris Halliday, D.D.S., M.P.H.
Larry Herman, D.M.D.
Kim Hort, D.M.D.
Mark Horton, O.D., M.D.
Laurie Hynes, R.D.H.
Ankur Kalra, O.D.

William Kohn, D.D.S.
Marsha Lambrou, R.N.
Chris Lamer, Pharm.D., C.D.E.
Donnie Lee, M.D.
Flora Lum, M.D.
Maria Matthews
Cheryl Metheny, M.S., R.D./L.D.N., C.D.E., C.L.C.
Kristin Nichols, Pharm.D.
Roland Palmquist, D.P.M.
Lauren Patton, D.D.S.
Dennis Pena, D.P.M.
Matthew Pettengill, D.P.M.
Meerah Ramesh, M.S., R.D., C.D.E.
Terry Raymer, M.D., C.D.E.
Stephen RithNajarian, M.D.
Thomas Rogers, D.D.S.
Jody Rosendahl, R.D.
Mark Rothstein, D.P.M., M.P.H.
Michael Schroeder, D.D.S.
Mark Sherstinsky, O.D.
Judith Thompson, Pharm.D., B.C.P.S.
Carol Treat, M.S., R.D., C.D.E., L.D.
Roger VanDyke, R.N.
Nicole Vesely

Contents

Foreword

The goals of *Working Together to Manage Diabetes: A Guide for Pharmacists, Podiatrists, Optometrists, and Dental Professionals* is to reinforce consistent diabetes messages across the four disciplines, pharmacy, podiatry, optometry, and dentistry (PPOD), and to promote a team approach to comprehensive diabetes care that encourages collaboration among all care providers.

The following are the learning objectives for these materials:
After this activity, the participant will be able to...

- Identify the ABCs of diabetes and their role in preventing complications.

- Name key messages that PPOD providers should all convey to patients with diabetes.

- Describe the key concerns for drug management and foot, eye, and oral health care for people with diabetes.

- Identify the results of the Diabetes Prevention Program (DPP).

The target audiences that may best benefit from these materials include pharmacists, podiatrists, optometrists, dentists, dental hygienists, physicians, nurses, dietitians, and others who provide care to people with or at risk for diabetes.

Working Together to Manage Diabetes is a cross-training document. It is not a comprehensive guide to all diabetes concerns in any one of the PPOD disciplines, but is instead a "key issues" guide to messages that every health care professional can give to support comprehensive care.

Hypothetical Case Examples

- A 70-year-old woman with diabetes tells her eye care provider that her blurred vision is such a problem that she is afraid to cut her toenails. She states "They are so long, my shoes don't fit!" She has worn oversized bedroom slippers to the appointment. The eye care provider asks the patient to take off her slippers, and finds overgrown, thickened toenails that have curled around and are cutting the skin. The woman has little sensation and has noticed no pain though several areas are red. The eye care provider arranges for the patient to be seen that day by her primary care provider or a podiatrist for foot care and emphasizes the importance of prompt treatment to avoid serious injury.

- A dental hygienist notes that her patient smokes. She tells him that smoking can cause oral cancer and she describes the impact tobacco use can have on increasing diabetes complications. She asks the patient to consider quitting as an important step in controlling his diabetes and gives him the 1-800-QUITNOW number.

- A 40-year-old woman asks her local pharmacist for advice on reading glasses. She says, "I must be getting older, everything is just blurry." The pharmacist uncovers a history of diabetes, diagnosed the previous year, but discovers that the patient never returned for follow-up. The pharmacist advises the woman that her blurred vision may not be a need for reading glasses but in fact a sign of diabetes and arranges for the woman to be seen by a primary care provider and eye care provider for follow-up.

- A podiatrist notices his 35-year-old patient with diabetes has terrible breath and asks about it. The patient is embarrassed but admits that he has noticed a bad taste as well. A quick look in the patient's mouth reveals inflamed, swollen gums with pus at the gum line. The podiatrist describes the link between periodontal disease and poor blood glucose control and stresses the need for urgent dental attention for a possible abscess. The podiatrist's office helps the patient obtain a same-day dental appointment for care.

- A dentist needs to schedule a patient for several procedures and asks about the timing of the patient's morning insulin. The patient is confused about his complicated medication regimen and asks, "Should I just skip all medicines that day until after you work on my teeth?" The dentist phones the patient's pharmacist to arrange a consultation. The pharmacist collaborates with the primary care clinician to develop an individualized medication schedule and advises the patient and his dentist on whether to hold medications the day of the procedure.

- A man with diabetes of more than 20 years duration, and neuropathy, asks the pharmacist for an Ace wrap and advice on care of his foot, which is warm, red, and swollen. The man recalls no trauma and there is no evidence of skin breakdown or an open wound. The pharmacist arranges for a same-day referral to a podiatrist for possible cellulitis. Upon physical exam and X ray of the affected foot, the podiatrist diagnoses Charcot arthropathy and implements a plan of treatment with no weight bearing and close follow-up, with casting, until the edema resolves.

Where can I ever find the time?

How realistic is it for a busy optometrist to look at a patient's feet? Or any of the scenarios described above? You have limited time to provide patient care. But research has shown that health messages direct from the provider, e.g., "I recommend that you..." are more effective than generalizations or third-person recommendations such as "You should see someone about that..." or "The American Diabetes Association says that..."

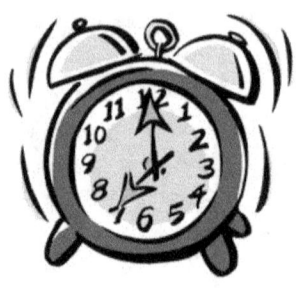

You don't need to be an expert or do a thorough exam to identify that a problem needs attention by a specialist. It takes less than a minute to look at a person's foot, mouth, or eye, or to ask a few questions about medications, supplies, or tobacco use. You reinforce the importance of preventive care if you take time to check a complaint yourself before recommending referral to another provider. Support comprehensive diabetes care: think beyond your own discipline to identify other potential problems. Then refer with an "I recommend..." message. Patients will appreciate your concern for their health and well-being as a whole. Establishing a referral system with other providers can improve your patient's health and increase your referral base as well.

Section 1

Diabetes: A Major Health Problem

Diabetes is a serious, common, costly, but controllable disease. Diabetes is the sixth leading cause of death in the United States and affects almost 21 million Americans, an estimated 6.2 million of whom are as yet undiagnosed (1). In 2002, diabetes cost the nation an estimated $132 billion in direct and indirect costs (2). Diabetes is the number one cause of lower limb amputation not related to trauma, the number one cause of acquired blindness, and the number one cause of kidney disease leading to dialysis in the United States. Diabetes is a major contributor to cardiovascular disease, the number one cause of death in this country. About 65% of people with diabetes die from cardiovascular disease (3).

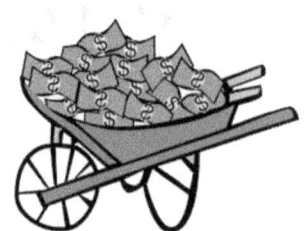

Diabetes Impact*
- Affects almost 21 million people in the United States.
- One third (more than 6 million people) are as yet undiagnosed.
- Costs more than $132 billion/year in health care expenditures.
- One of the six leading causes of death in the United States.
- Number 1 cause of acquired blindness.
- Number 1 cause of kidney failure.
- Number 1 cause of non-traumatic amputation.
- Major contributor to cardiovascular disease, the #1 cause of death.

* Source: 2005 Diabetes Fact Sheet

Diabetes prevalence is rapidly increasing. Figure 1 shows self-reported rates of diabetes gathered through the Behavioral Risk Factor Surveillance Study (BRFSS) by state. Diabetes prevalence has tripled from 1990 to 2005, and in some states more than 25% of the adult population aged 20 years and older has diabetes. The number of people with diabetes in the United States is projected to reach 39 million by the year 2050 (4). If current trends continue, 1 in 3 Americans will develop diabetes sometime in his or her lifetime, and those with diabetes will lose, on average, 10 to 15 years of life (5).

Types of Diabetes

Type 1 diabetes. Type 1 diabetes (formerly known as insulin-dependent or juvenile-onset diabetes) is an autoimmune disease that is distinguished by the destruction of insulin-producing beta cells. Type 1 diabetes can occur at any age, but onset usually begins in childhood or the young adult years. People with type 1 diabetes are ketosis-prone, although ketoacidosis can develop in type 2 diabetes as well. People with type 1 diabetes must take insulin daily. Delivery mechanisms for insulin include injection, insulin pump, and inhalation, although at this time inhalation must be combined with another delivery method. For optimal management, people with type 1 diabetes must test their blood glucose levels several times a day, follow an individualized meal plan, and engage in regular physical activity.

Type 2 diabetes. Formerly known as non-insulin-dependent or adult-onset diabetes, type 2 diabetes is related to insulin resistance. The pancreas continues to make insulin, but the insulin is not used well by other body tissues. Eventually, insulin production decreases. People with type 2 diabetes may be treated with insulin, oral medications, or a combination of both or be controlled with a food plan and physical activity alone. Type 2 diabetes affects 9.6% of the U.S. population aged 20 years and older, and 20.9% of the population aged 60 years or more, occurring more often in adults who are overweight and sedentary (3). In recent years, however, it has been seen increasingly in young people, including children. The prevalence of type 2 diabetes in younger age groups is of special concern because the risk of complications increases with the disease's duration.

Type 2 diabetes disproportionately affects African Americans, Hispanics/Latinos, American Indians, and Alaska Natives, and some groups of Asians and Native Hawaiians or other Pacific Islanders. African Americans and Hispanic/Latino Americans are about twice as likely to have diabetes as non-Hispanic/Latino whites in a similar age group. Some populations of American Indians have the highest rates of diabetes in the world.

Gestational diabetes is a form of glucose intolerance diagnosed in some women during pregnancy. Gestational diabetes occurs more frequently among African Americans, Hispanic/Latino Americans, and American Indians. It is also more common among obese women and those with a family history of diabetes. During pregnancy, gestational diabetes requires treatment to normalize maternal blood glucose levels to avoid complications in the infant. After pregnancy, 5% to 10% of women with gestational diabetes are found to have type 2 diabetes. Women who have had gestational diabetes have a 20% to 50% chance of developing diabetes in the next 5 to 10 years (5).

Other types of diabetes result from specific genetic conditions (such as maturity-onset diabetes of youth), surgery, drugs, malnutrition, infections, and other illnesses. Such types of diabetes account for 1% to 5% of all diagnosed cases.

Diabetes and Obesity Trends

The development of type 2 diabetes is multifactorial, with insulin resistance, sedentary lifestyle, increasing age and increasing obesity contributing to this increase. A body mass index (BMI) of 25 or more (> 23 for Asian Americans and > 26 for Pacific Islanders) is a risk factor for the development of type 2 diabetes. Figure 2 shows the parallel increases in the prevalence of diabetes and mean body weight by year in the United States from 1990 to 2000 (6–8). As of 2005, approximately two-thirds of American adults were overweight or obese, with BMI more than 25.

- The prevalence of obesity has increased by 61% since 1991.
- More than 60% of U.S. adults are overweight.
- BMI and weight gain are major risk factors for diabetes.

Figure 1. Diabetes and Obesity Trends in the United States

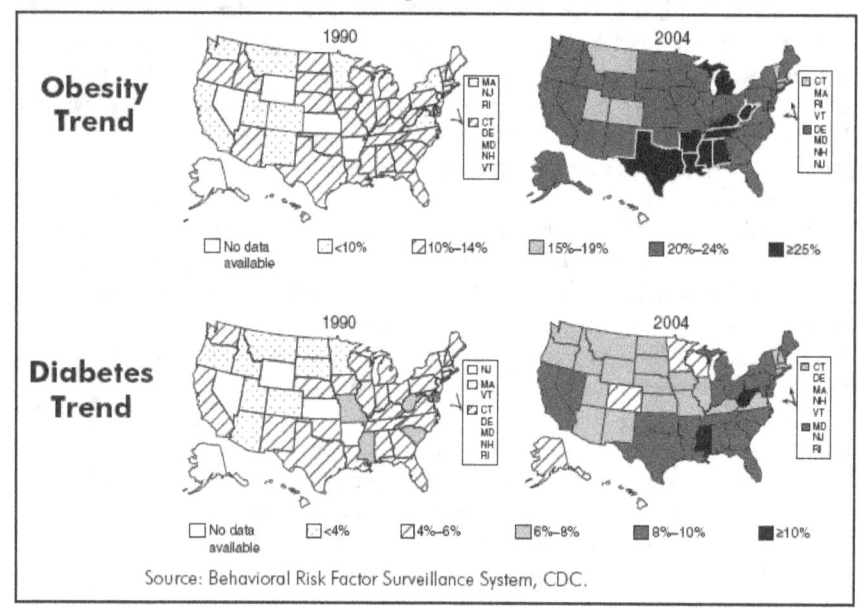

Figure 2. Diabetes and Obesity

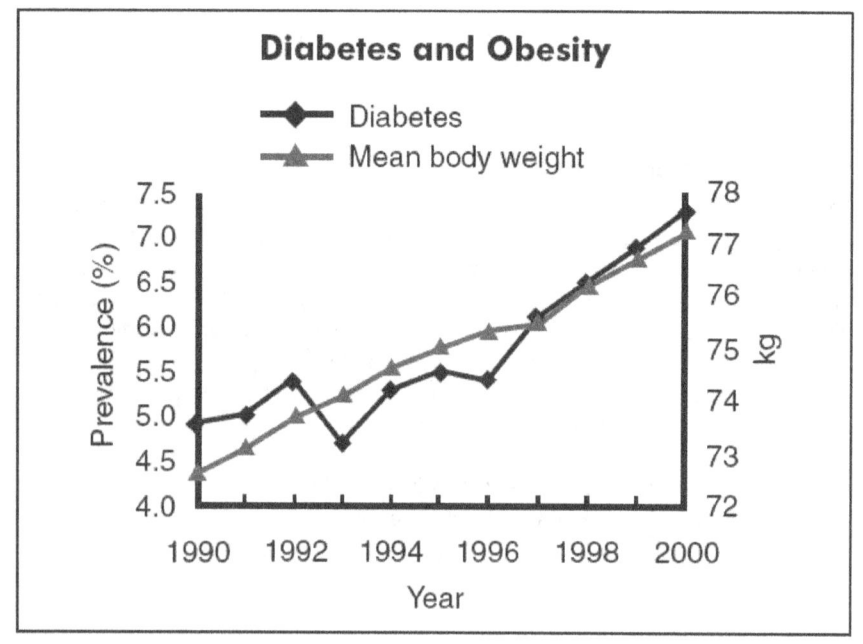

Diabetes Morbidity and Mortality

Adults with type 2 diabetes are two to four times more likely to have heart disease or suffer a stroke than those without diabetes. Cardiovascular disease is the major cause of death for people with diabetes. They are also at risk for other complications, such as blindness, kidney disease, amputations, nervous system disease, and oral complications, including gum or periodontal disease and tooth loss (3).

Fortunately, many studies in recent years have demonstrated effective interventions to help prevent or delay diabetes complications as well as the disease itself (9–21).

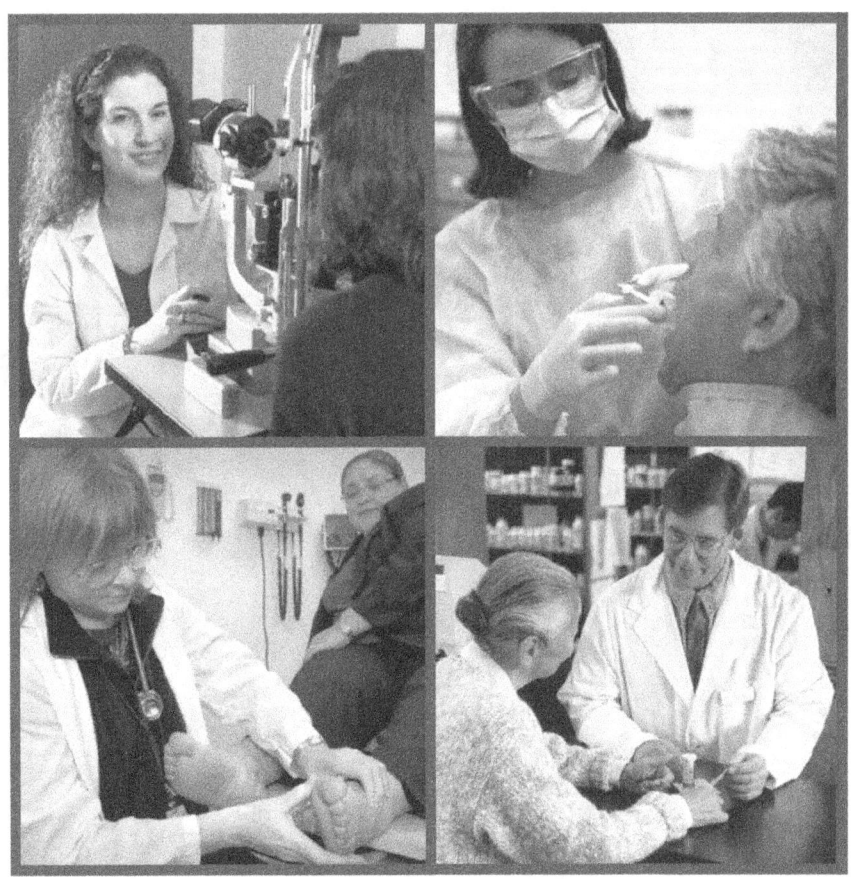

Section 2

Impact of Controlling the ABCs of Diabetes

Impact of glycemic control

Table 1 summarizes some of the major studies that have demonstrated the impact of glycemic control on complications prevention. The Diabetes Control and Complications Trial (DCCT) showed that tight glycemic control reduced risk of microvascular disease in persons with type 1 diabetes (76% reduction in eye disease overall with 63% reduction in retinopathy, 54% reduction in nephropathy, 60% reduction in neuropathy) (9, 10). The United Kingdom Prospective Diabetes Study (UKPDS) showed that among people with type 2 diabetes, improved glycemic control (average A1c = 7% vs. average A1c = 7.9% in the conventionally treated group) led to a reduction in risk of 25% for microvascular disease overall, 17%–21% for retinopathy, and 24%–33% for albuminuria. Lower A1c values also reduced the incidence of macrovascular disease with a 16% reduction in myocardial infarction, and contributed to a 24% decrease in cataract extraction (12).

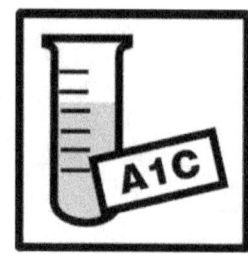

Table 1. Impact of Glycemic Control (9–11, 26)

Good Glycemic Control (Lower A1C) Reduces Incidence of Complications		
	DCCT	UKPDS
A1C	9➔7	8➔7
Retinopathy	63%	17–21%
Neuropathy	54%	24–33%
Nephropathy	60%	—
Macrovascular		
Disease	41%†	16%†

† Not statistically significant

Impact of Blood Pressure Control

The United Kingdom Prospective Diabetes Study (UKPDS) found that improved glycemic control not only reduced diabetes complications, but also demonstrated the impact of improved blood pressure control. UKPDS participants in the "tight" control blood pressure group maintained on average for the duration of the study 10 mm Hg lower systolic and 5 mm Hg lower diastolic pressures than controls. Table 2 summarizes the impact of that reduction. Improved blood pressure control (average of 144/82 mm Hg vs. 154/87 mm Hg control) during the 8 years led to a reduction in risk of 34% for retinopathy, 47% for vision loss, 37% overall for microvascular disease, 56% for heart failure, and 44% for stroke incidence (12).

Table 2. UKPDS: Impact of Blood Pressure Control in Diabetes (12)

Tight blood pressure control reduces risk of:
• Retinopathy progression (34%)
• Vision loss (47%)
• Diabetes-related deaths (32%)
• Microvascular disease (37%)
• Heart failure (56%)
• Stroke (44%)

UK Prospective Diabetes Study Group (UKPDS) 33: Lancet. 1998; 352: 837-853.

Furthermore, clinical trials, such as ABCD (Appropriate Blood Pressure Control in Diabetes Trial) and HOPE (Heart Outcomes Prevention Evaluation Study), also show that use of an ACE inhibitor reduces the risk of heart attack, stroke, or cardiovascular death by 25%–30% in patients with type 2 diabetes, and slows the progression of the kidney damage of diabetes (14).

Impact of Cholesterol and Other Lipid Control

Among people with diabetes, 67% have one or more lipid abnormalities. Multiple studies, including CARE (Cholesterol and Recurrent Events Trial) and 4S (Scandinavian Simvastatin Survival Study), have shown that lipid therapy can reduce the risk of coronary events such as nonfatal heart attacks and CVD-related deaths, as summarized in Table 3 (13, 19).

Table 3. CARE and 4S: Impact of Cholesterol Control in Diabetes

Lipid therapy reduces risk of coronary events
Cholesterol and Recurrent Events Trail (CARE) Reduced risk by 24%
Scandinavian Simvastatin Survival Study (4S) Reduced risk by 42% to 55%

Preventing Complications

Comprehensive diabetes care is a team effort involving self-management behaviors (see "Self-Management Support" at the end of this section) by the patient and preventive care services by health care providers. At routine visits, providers of foot, dental, and eye care and drug therapy management can monitor, prevent, and treat complications, not only for conditions specific to their professional discipline, but for the patient's overall health. Cardiovascular disease (CVD), including heart disease and stroke, is the number one cause of death for people with diabetes. All health care providers can contribute to the reduction of risk factors for CVD, and potentially reduce other complications as well, by reinforcing control of the ABCs of diabetes:

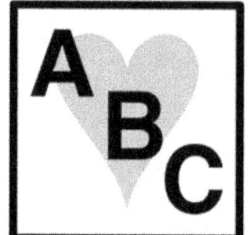

Treatment Goals for the ABCs of Diabetes
A1C < 7 %
Preprandial plasma glucose 90–130 mg/dl
Peak postprandial plasma glucose < 180 mg/dl
(usually 1 to 2 hours after the start of a meal)
Blood pressure (mmHg)
Systolic Diastolic
< 130 / < 80
Cholesterol – Lipid Profile (mg/dl)
LDL Cholesterol < 100
HDL Cholesterol Men > 40 Women > 50
Triglycerides < 150

Individualize Treatment Goals
For example, consider:
- A1C goal as close to normal (< 6%) as possible without significant hypoglycemia.
- Less stringent AIC goal for people with severe or frequent hypoglycemia.
- Lower blood pressure goals for people with nephropathy.

The NDEP promotes control of the ABCs of diabetes and use of the term A1C for Hemoglobin A1c.

Source: Numbers At A Glance www.ndep.nih.gov

A **is for A1C**, previously known as hemoglobin A1C—a test that reflects average blood glucose over the last 3 months. The goal for most people with diabetes is <7. An A1C of 7 corresponds to an average blood glucose level of 150 mg/dL.

B **is for blood pressure.** The goal for most people with diabetes is <130/80 mm Hg.

C **is for cholesterol.** The goal for people with diabetes is an LDL level of <100 mg/dL, an HDL level of >40 mg/dl in men and >50 in women, and triglycerides level of <150

Source: American Diabetes Association Standards of Medical Care, Diabetes Care 29 (Suppl.1): S4-S42, 2006 (27).

Section 3

Diabetes Management and Team Care

Diabetes Management And Team Care

People with diabetes can take action to lower their risk for heart attack, stroke, and other diabetes complications by controlling the ABCs, following an individualized meal plan, engaging in regular physical activity, avoiding tobacco use, and taking medicines as prescribed. A multidisciplinary team approach is critical to success in diabetes care and complications prevention. Medical nutrition therapy education by a dietitian is critical to developing an individualized meal plan. A certified diabetes educator not only teaches factual information about diabetes but also provides self-management support, enabling the patient to gain skills in problem solving and self-care. All health care providers can help by discussing how self-management and diabetes control relate to preventing complications.

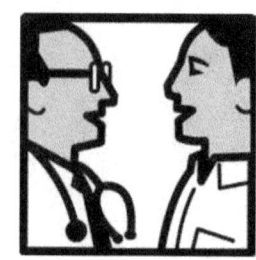

Tools for health care providers and patients can be found on the NDEP Web site at http://ndep.nih.gov/. The NDEP Team Care monograph, available at http://ndep.nih.gov/diabetes/pubs/TeamCare.pdf (28), can tell you more about the advantages of team care and how to form a team, and gives examples of effective team care. For information on the link between diabetes and cardiovascular disease, see http://ndep.nih.gov/control/cvd.htm.

Self-management Support

Patient self-management support is important in helping people achieve goals in both diabetes control and prevention. In contrast to traditional patient education, in which information is delivered to the person with diabetes, self-management support involves teaching the behavioral skills needed to make decisions about diabetes management in daily life. Self-management support is a partnership between patient and health care provider. It involves collaborative goal-setting, problem-solving, and individualized behavior-change plans that address concerns identified by the patient as highest priority. All health care providers can provide self-management support, reinforcing patient problem-solving skills and giving consistent, proactive health care messages.

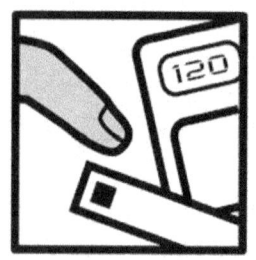

Self-management support relies on principles of self-efficacy (confidence in one's ability to perform a task successfully), short-term action plans, realistic goal setting, and proactive identification of barriers to optimal diabetes control. Self-management support involves asking the person with diabetes to identify an accomplishable action he or she would like to take in changing a behavior (e.g., walking 10 minutes a day before dinner starting tomorrow), not telling the individual what to do. Self-management support also includes trouble-shooting about missed appointments, establishing routines around daily activities such as dental hygiene, foot care or blood glucose testing, and helping people overcome the barriers to receiving regular screening exams for eye, foot and oral health.

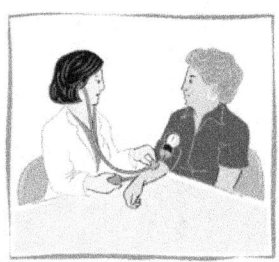

Self-Management Support

At each visit, the provider and patient need to consider the following patient self-management tasks. How to:

- Take care of diabetes and it's complications.

- Incorporate behavior changes into daily life activities.

- Manage emotions, including future concerns.

Source: http://www.betterdiabetescare.nih.gov/WHATpatientcentereddimensions.htm.

Self-management support does not replace traditional patient education but complements it. Because diet and physical activity patterns are important in both diabetes control and prevention, it is important that all providers participate in patient self-management support for healthy food choices and regular exercise. Prompting a patient to consider and plan for challenging events is self-management support. Problem solving discussions can help prepare the patient to deal effectively with self-management issues.

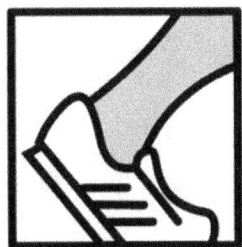

Self-management Support Example

A 50-year-old man with diabetes and obesity has been told he would benefit from a less calorie-dense diet, but he confesses to you that he just doesn't think he can do it. You are not a dietitian—how can you help him make such a change?

- Ask what he thinks will be the biggest challenge to making these changes.

- Ask if he can identify one thing he can do differently.

- Reinforce all positive steps, even if small.

- Refer him to a dietitian or diabetes educator who can continue support.

- Follow up at the next visit by asking about progress.

In this example, the man might identify eating dessert as a challenge, and a change in portion size (e.g., eating one scoop of ice cream instead of two) as one thing he can do differently. This is an acceptable short-term goal. It is a step in the right direction. All health care providers can contribute to self-management support by helping patients plan and troubleshoot the many daily decisions they must make for diabetes control.

Self-management support also involves follow up: asking about progress in achieving behavioral goals and sustaining problem-solving skills (29). To learn more about self-management support, consult the NDEP's Better Diabetes Care Web site www.betterdiabetescare.nih.gov.

Psychosocial considerations and comorbid conditions such as depression can adversely influence self-management behaviors. Multi-disciplinary team care includes working closely with social services, certified diabetes educators, and mental health specialists who can help address these concerns. More information can be found in the NDEP Team Care monograph available at http://ndep.nih.gov as well as at www.betterdiabetescare.nih.gov.

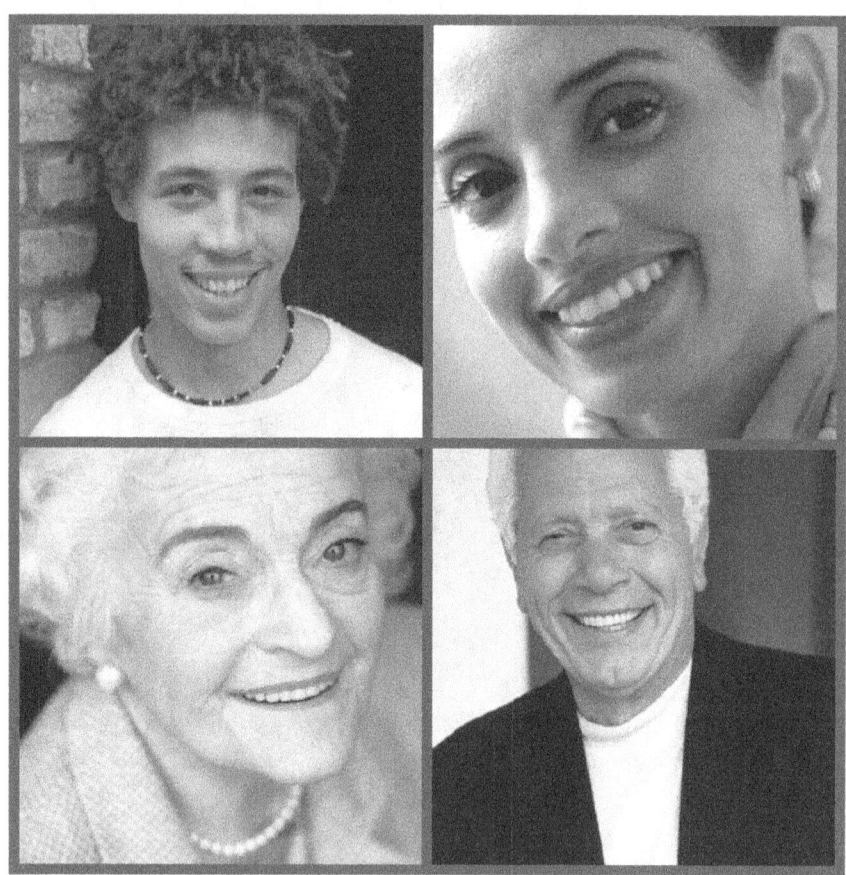

Section 4

**What to Dicuss with Patients
with Diabetes**

What to Discuss with Patients with Diabetes

This section provides messages that you as a health care provider should discuss with people with diabetes about foot, eye, and oral health and about drug therapy management. The bullets highlight questions to ask and information to discuss about diabetes-associated risks, the benefits of comprehensive care, the need for regular medical examinations, symptoms to look for, and self-care issues. You can discuss these topics, when appropriate, over a series of patient visits; you need not cover all the material with every patient. Guidelines for referral to other health care providers are also provided.

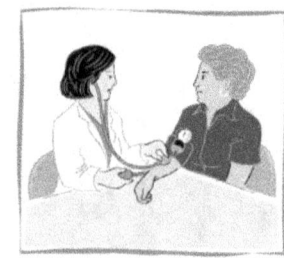

Key Messages all Health Care Providers Can Reinforce

- Emphasize the importance of metabolic control (ABCs).

- Promote a healthy lifestyle.

- Explain the benefits of diabetes comprehensive team care.

- Recommend routine exams for complication prevention: oral health, comprehensive foot exam, complete dilated eye exam.

- Reinforce self-exams.

- Recognize danger signs and seek help.

- Promote pharmacist role in drug therapy management.

Promote the ABCs—A1C, Blood Pressure, and Cholesterol

It is important to control risk factors for cardiovascular disease. Ask about the ABCs of diabetes.

- **Ask:** "Do you know your ABC goals and how to reach them?" Recommend working with the health care team to determine both long-and short-term goals for each ABC.

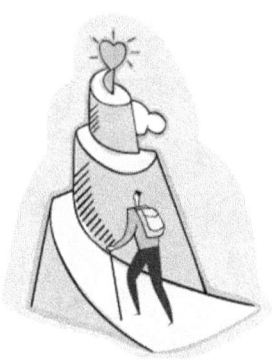

- **Advise:** "You can take action to prevent or delay type 2 diabetes complications." Controlling the ABCs can reduce the risk for heart attack and stroke, and inform them that poor control can lead to problems in foot, eye, and oral health. Explain that screening and team care can prevent complications.

- **Assist:** Refer to a primary care provider. Give your patients resources to help them make healthy changes by contacting the National Diabetes Education Program (NDEP) for FREE information and materials on diabetes prevention and control. Recommend that they call 1-800-438-5383 or visit www.ndep.nih.gov.

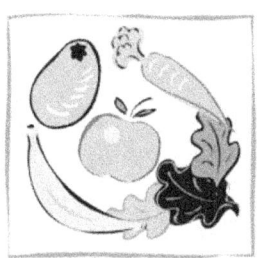

Promote a Healthy Lifestyle

Healthy lifestyle is key to diabetes control.

- **Weight.** Advise people with diabetes to aim for a healthy weight. Emphasize the importance of setting stepwise and realistic goals for weight reduction.

- **Healthy Food Choices.** Encourage meal planning that includes a variety of foods and controls portion sizes and snacks. Increasing fiber and limiting saturated fats and salts will help control blood glucose, blood pressure, and cholesterol. Recommend consultation with a dietitian for additional help with meal planning and learning how to make healthy food choices.

- **Physical activity.** Advise people with diabetes that moderate physical activity (such as walking) can help control the ABCs and prevent complications.

- **Self-management.** Ask people with diabetes to identify their high priority concerns. Prompt them to plan for challenging situations and set short-term achievable goals. Compliment them on any steps taken toward these goals. See "Self-Management Support" in the previous section.

- **Tobacco.** Ask about tobacco use. Encourage people with diabetes to avoid smoking and using smokeless tobacco products. Recommend calling the FREE tobacco quit line 1-800-QUITNOW. People who use tobacco are at greater risk for stroke; heart, kidney, and eye diseases; nerve damage; and lower-extremity complications. To learn more about tobacco cessation strategies, consult the CDC's Tobacco Information and Prevention Source (TIPS) Web site at www.cdc.gov/tobacco/.

Explain the Risks of Disease and Benefits of Care

People with diabetes make daily decisions that affect their diabetes control. Cornerstones of diabetes self management include meal planning, physical activity, and self monitoring of blood glucose. Routine self-care behaviors also impact diabetes complications prevention. See appendix C for a list of common diabetes-related foot, eye, and oral health complaints and examples of inappropriate self-care.

At each patient encounter, remind patients of the risks of diabetes complications and the benefits of foot, eye, and oral health care as well as drug therapy management. Ask about annual screening exams. Ask about routine self-care behaviors. Assess symptoms that warrant urgent referral.

- **Foot health.** Ask people with diabetes if they know how diabetes affects their feet. Explain that diabetes raises the risk of foot ulcers, which can lead to amputation, and that proper foot care reduces their risk.

  - **Foot exams.** Ask people with diabetes if they have had a comprehensive foot examination (including a sensory exam with a monofilament) in the past year. Recommend a comprehensive annual foot exam by a podiatric physician or primary care clinician and a foot inspection (visual foot check) at every primary care provider visit.

- **Daily foot care.** Ask about proper daily foot care. People with neuropathy may not notice injuries as they do not feel pain. Advise all people with diabetes to take the following steps:

  - Examine feet daily, both by looking and touching. Look for cuts, bruises, puncture wounds, corns or calluses, areas of redness, or pus. Seek podiatric medical advice right away for these symptoms.

  - Clean feet (both skin and nails) daily and dry the spaces between the toes gently. Check the insides of shoes for objects before putting them on.

  - Never walk barefoot, not even indoors. Wear appropriate footwear, such as athletic or walking shoes that fit well and cover the feet (i.e., NOT sandals).

  - Foot symptoms. Ask about foot symptoms and recommend prompt podiatric medical attention for bruises, lacerations, puncture wounds, swelling, and areas of redness or pus from any area of the foot. These signs and symptoms can be the earliest harbingers of serious injury leading to amputation. Be proactive.

  - Refer people with these symptoms to a podiatric physician or to their primary care provider.

- **Eye health.** Advise people with diabetes about the risk of diabetic retinopathy, a leading cause of blindness in adults and one that may be prevented or delayed by good control of blood glucose. People with diabetes also may be at greater risk for eye problems such as cataracts and glaucoma. Ocular symptoms associated with diabetes include fluctuation in visual acuity, double vision, dry eye, recurrent lid infections (blepharitis) and changes in color vision.

  - **Eye exams.** Ask when the person with diabetes last had a comprehensive dilated eye exam by an optometrist or an ophthalmologist. Reinforce the need for regular screening eye exams to prevent or delay the onset of blindness due to diabetic retinopathy. Most people with diabetes should have a dilated eye examination by an optometrist or an ophthalmologist annually. An eye care provider may suggest less frequent exams (every 2–3 years) in the setting of a normal eye exam (30). Examinations will be needed more frequently if retinopathy exists or is progressing.

  - **Eye care.** Advise people with diabetes to report eye symptoms to their health care provider and to maintain a current prescription for eyeglasses, contact lenses, or low-vision aids.

  - **Eye symptoms.** Ask about eye symptoms and their frequency and duration. Encourage people with diabetes to report any changes in their eyes or vision, such as sudden onset of blurriness, seeing spots, or persistent redness or pain to their health care provider.
    - If there is sudden change in vision, refer the person at once to an optometrist or ophthalmologist.

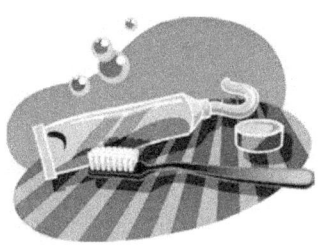

- **Oral health.** Explain the link between poor control of blood glucose and periodontal (gum) disease. Good oral health may help control diabetes— and controlling blood glucose levels my contribute to improved oral health.

  - **Oral health exams.** Ask the date of the last dental/oral health exam. Stress the importance of good oral hygiene and regular exams, including regular cleanings performed by a dental hygienist or dentist to prevent periodontal disease. Even people with who wear dentures or have no teeth need an oral health exam once a year to screen for cancer, infection, or other lesions.

  - **Daily oral care.** Advise about the need to brush the teeth after eating and to floss at least once a day. If dentures are worn, advise about their care: daily cleaning and a dental visit if dentures become loose or irritation develops.

  - **Monthly oral self exam.** Advise people with diabetes to do a monthly self exam and to contact their dentist if they notice signs of infection, such as sore, swollen, or bleeding gums; loose teeth; or mouth ulcers.

  - **Oral symptoms.** Ask about oral health symptoms that may indicate infection such as a bad taste or bad breath, or pain. Evaluate whether an acute problem, such as infection, is present that requires immediate attention.

    - **Refer** individuals with oral findings or complaints to a dentist or periodontist and/or their primary care provider, as indicated.

    - Oral infections may worsen glycemic control, progress to serious complications quickly, and need prompt treatment.

- **Drug therapy management.** Discuss the benefits of proper drug therapy management. Recommend that your patients with diabetes talk with their pharmacist about how to get the most benefit from medications by individualizing dosage regimens. Pharmacists can provide regular medication reviews to ensure that people with diabetes take medications as prescribed and understand the risks of using over-the-counter (OTC) medications.

- **Regular Medication Review.** Advise people with diabetes that regular medication reviews, individualized drug regimens, and screening for interactions and side effects from medications, OTC medications, herbal products, and supplements can help them get the most from their drug therapy.

  - **Medications.** Ask people with diabetes if they take their medication exactly as prescribed. Advise them to talk to their pharmacist or primary care provider if they are unable to follow the medication plan prescribed.

    - Remind people with diabetes that they should seek advice from their pharmacist or primary care provider before taking any OTC medications, herbal products, or other supplements.

- **Drug Therapy Management Medication**-related symptoms.

  - Ask at every visit about medication use.

  - Ask people with diabetes to report any changes in symptoms, medical conditions, medications, doses, supplements, or lifestyle to all health care providers.

  - Refer individuals to a pharmacist or primary care provider, as indicated, for evaluation.

- **Selection and use of a blood glucose meter.** Refer people with diabetes to a pharmacist or diabetes educator for help in choosing an appropriate blood glucose meter, learning how to use it, and understanding the results to check how medications are working.

- **ABC monitoring.** Ask your patients with diabetes when they last had their A1C, blood pressure, and cholesterol levels checked and if they know the results of these tests.

- **Personal ABCs.** Ask if they know what they need to do to control their ABCs. Advise about the ABC goals: A1C <7, BP <130/80, LDL cholesterol <100. Even if a person has not reached these goals, there is benefit in decreasing their A1C, blood pressure, and cholesterol towards these goals.

How can a busy health care provider find the time to give the key team care messages?

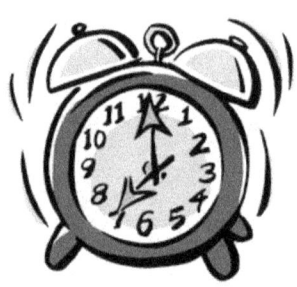

Suggestions:

- Don't give every message at one appointment.

- Customize and prioritize messages according to the patient's needs.

- Establish a blueprint of messages over a period of client appointments.

- Provide patient with a computer generated reminder of key messages discussed at each appointment.

- Document what is accomplished at each appointment and the patient's response.

- Create pamphlets for office or use NDEP materials.

- Include key messages in office newsletters.

- Offer health awareness program for patients with diabetes.

- Establish referral base in the community.

Table 4. Summary—What to Discuss with Patients with Diabetes

This table outlines messages that health care providers should discuss with people who have diabetes regarding foot, eye, and oral health and about drug therapy management.

Health care providers in these four disciplines are well positioned to deliver these overarching prevention messages, communicate the need for metabolic control, and encourage multidisciplinary team diabetes control.

Promote the ABCs—A1C, Blood Pressure, and Cholesterol:	Ask about Health Examinations:
– Controlling the ABCs can prevent complications and reduce the risk of stroke and heart attack.	– Foot exams.
– Ask: "Do you know your ABC goals and how to reach them?"	– Eye exams.
– Explain that poor ABC control can also lead to problems in foot, eye, and oral health.	– Oral health exams.
	– Drug therapy management.
Promote a Healthy Lifestyle:	– ABC monitoring and control.
– Weight control.	
– Healthy food choices.	**Support Self-Care Behaviors:**
– Daily physical activity.	– Daily foot care.
– Support self management.	– Eye care.
– No tobacco use (call 1-800-QUITNOW for help).	– Daily oral care.
	– Monthly oral self-exam.
Explain the Risks and Benefits of Diabetes Comprehensive Control:	– Selection and use of a blood glucose monitor.
– Foot health.	– Know your ABC goals and how to reach them.
– Eye health.	– Medication management.
– Oral health.	
– Drug therapy management.	**Assess Symptoms that Require Referral:**
	– Foot symptoms.
	– Eye symptoms.
	– Oral symptoms.
	– Medication-related symptoms.

Table 5. Summary—What to Discuss with Patients with Diabetes

The information below lists some of the common issues specific to foot, eye, and oral health, and drug therapy management.

When health care professionals understand the diabetes care issues of other disciplines, they can recognize symptomatic concerns warranting urgent referral, reinforce annual screening recommendations, and contribute to a proactive approach to diabetes care beyond the scope of their particular discipline.

Foot Health	Eye Health	Oral Health	Drug Therapy Management
Diabetes-Related Foot Conditions:	Diabetes-Related Eye Conditions:	Diabetes-Related Oral Health Conditions:	Diabetes drug management issues:
– Neuropathy	– Retinopathy	– Changes in the oral cavity	– Improper drug choice
– Vasculopathy	– Double vision	– Periodontal disease	– Underdosage
– Dermatological conditions	– Vision fluctuations	– Oral Candida (thrush)	– Overdosage
– Musculoskeletal problems	– Cataracts		– Adverse drug reactions
	– Macular edema		– Drug interactions
	– Ocular nerve palsy		– Undertreatment
Comprehensive Foot Examination to identify the high-risk foot:	Comprehensive Eye Examination:	Comprehensive Oral Examination:	Strategies for Managing Drug Therapy:
– Loss of protective sensation	– Visual acuity	– Teeth	– Use of medications
– Skin and nail condition	– Visual fields	– Gums	– Monitoring treatment
– Absent pedal pulses	– Pupillary reaction	– Periodontal probing	– Self treatment and OTC medications
– Foot deformity	– Intraocular pressure	– Intraoral lesions, infections, or masses	– Selecting and using a blood glucose meter
– History of foot ulcers	– Cranial nerves	– Adequate saliva flow	– Cost control
– Prior amputation	– Slit-lamp exam		
	– Dilated retinal exam		Coordination of Care

Section 5

Foot Health and Diabetes

Foot Health and Diabetes

Prevalence of Foot Symptoms and Complications

Early manifestations of diabetes may present initially in the foot. Foot symptoms increase the risk for co-morbid complications, of which non-traumatic lower-extremity amputations (LEAs) are the greatest concern. According to 1997 hospital discharge data, diabetes accounted for approximately 87,720 LEAs in the United States, fully 67% of all LEAs (31). Between 1980 and 2001, the number of diabetes-related hospital discharges with LEA increased from an average of 33,000 to 82,000 per year (32). LEA rates were highest among men, non-Hispanics/Latinos, African Americans, and the elderly. In 2003, there were about 75,000 diabetes-related hospital discharges with LEA. The LEA rate per 1,000 persons with diabetes that year was 3.9 among persons aged less than 65 years, 6.6 among persons aged 65–74 years, and 7.9 among persons aged 75 years or older.

One study found that 80% of non-traumatic LEAs are preceded by a foot ulceration, which provides a portal for infection (33). According to Behavioral Risk Factor Surveillance Study (BRFSS) data, approximately 12% of U.S. adults with diabetes had a history of foot ulcer, a risk factor for LEA (34). Another report identified minor trauma, ulceration, and faulty wound healing as precursors to 73% of LEAs, often in combination with gangrene and infection (37). Other risk factors include the presence of sensory peripheral neuropathy, altered biomechanics, elevated pressure on the sole of the foot, and limited joint mobility (35).

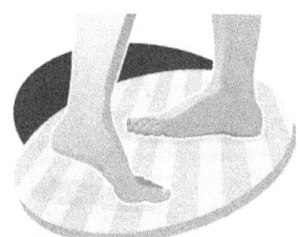

The Charcot Foot

Patients with neuropathy are at risk for painless degenerative arthropathy that typically affects the tarsometatarsal and metatarsophalangeal joints, resulting in a red, swollen, and possibly deformed foot that can be mistaken for cellulitis. Radiographs may show collapse of joint structure, and can be misinterpreted as osteomyelitis. Treatment for Charcot arthropathy, however, is not antibiotics but a non-weight-bearing cast (once any acute edema has resolved) and special shoes to correct altered biomechanics. Without proper treatment, the Charcot foot can progress to further deformity, ulceration and lead ultimately to amputation.

Consider it a "red flag" when a patient complains that his shoes no longer fit, or is wearing slippers or shoes with sections cut out to accommodate changes in foot shape, or walks with a new limp. A Charcot foot usually causes little to no pain and may be slowly progressive over weeks to months before coming to a foot care provider's attention. All health care providers can contribute to amputation prevention by referring patients with these signs and symptoms to a foot care specialist.

People with diabetes who have neuropathy are 1.7 times more likely to develop foot ulceration; in persons with both neuropathy and foot deformity, the risk is 12 times greater; and in those who also have a history of pathology (prior amputation or ulceration), the risk is 36 times greater (36, 37). Factors that increase risk for lower-extremity ulceration and amputation are male sex, the existence of diabetes for more than 10 years, tobacco use, a history of poor glycemic control, or the presence of cardiac, retinal, or renal complications (38–40).

Foot Complication Prevention

– Up to 20% of people with diabetes who present for routine care will have a treatable foot care problem. Have the patient remove socks and shoes and inspect both feet for acute problems at each visit.

– The lifetime incidence of foot ulcers among patients with diabetes is 15%. Most of these are preventable though interventions available in most primary care settings.

– Patients with diabetes on dialysis are at extreme risk for foot complications. Foot care programs that provide outreach to this group are associated with improved foot outcomes.

Foot Evaluation in People with Diabetes

Podiatrists use the following considerations to assess the risk for complications when evaluating the feet of people with diabetes.

- **Neuropathy.** The presence of subjective tingling, burning, numbness, or the sensation of bugs crawling on the skin may indicate peripheral sensory neuropathy. On clinical examination, this condition can be detected with an instrument known as a Semmes-Weinstein 5.07 (10 gram) monofilament. A description of how to use this monofilament to perform a comprehensive foot exam can be found in the free NDEP health care provider kit, Feet Can Last A Lifetime, http://www.ndep.nih.gov/diabetes/pubs/Feet_Kit_Eng.pdf.

- **Vasculopathy.** Cramping of calf muscles when walking ("charley horse") that requires frequent rest periods suggests intermittent claudication. This condition, often caused by insufficient blood supply to the region beneath the knee, indicates the presence of early or moderate occlusion of the arteries that is common to the lower extremities of people with diabetes. Intense cramping and aching in the toes only at night, called "rest pain," is usually relieved by hanging the feet over the side of the bed and by walking. This symptom signifies the end-stage blood vessel disorder and tissue ischemia that precedes diabetic gangrene. Although most clinical research continues to list the loss of sensation/neuropathy as the leading factor in ulceration and associated complications, poor blood supply can contribute to poor ulceration healing and is a significant risk factor for amputation. Both factors need to be addressed in comprehensive diabetes foot care with diagnostic testing for treatable vascular lesions and intervention as warranted.

- **Dermatological conditions.** Corns and calluses (hyperkeratotic lesions) of the feet result from elevated mechanical pressure and shearing of the skin. They often precede breakdown of skin and lead to blisters or ulceration. Superficial lacerations and heel fissures, or maceration (softening caused by wetness) between the toes, can all serve as portals for infection. Corns, calluses, toenail deformity, and bleeding beneath the nail may signify the presence of sensory neuropathy. Fungus infections of skin or nails can lead to secondary bacterial infections and should be treated.

- **Musculoskeletal symptoms.** Structural changes in the diabetic foot may develop in combination with muscle-tendon imbalances as a result of motor neuropathy. These deformities include the presence of hammertoes, bunions, high-arched foot, or flatfoot—all of which increase the potential for focal irritation of the foot in the shoe.

- **Lifestyle and family history.** People with diabetes who smoke are four times more likely than non-diabetic smokers to develop lower-extremity vascular disease. Unhealthy food choices and low physical activity levels contribute to poor long-term control of blood glucose and increase the risk that peripheral nervous system and/or blood vessel disorders will progress. A family history of cerebrovascular accidents and coronary artery disease may indicate a further increased risk of developing lower-extremity arterial complications. Inherited foot types (e.g., shapes) may predispose to biomechanical deformities that lead to problems with skin breakdown.

Comprehensive Foot Examination

A comprehensive foot examination for abnormalities, including evaluation of pulses, sensation, foot biomechanics (general foot structure and function), and nails helps determine the person's category of risk for developing foot complications. Persons with diabetes who are at high risk have one or more of the following characteristics: (1) loss of protective sensation, (2) absent pedal pulses, (3) foot deformity, (4) history of foot ulcers, or (5) prior amputation. Low-risk individuals have none of these characteristics (41). Assessment of risk status identifies people who need more intensive care and evaluation. Further patient education, early intervention, and special footwear if indicated can prevent ulcers and ultimately LEAs.

Patient Education

The goal for low-risk patients is to keep them at low risk through control of the ABCs and tobacco cessation in those who use tobacco. In high-risk patients, the goal is to prevent ulcers though self-management education, podiatry care, and proper use of appropriate footwear. Minor trauma, such as stubbing a toe or stepping on a sharp object, is the most frequent precipitating event leading to ulcer. Emphasize to patients and their families the need to be diligent in clearing the walking spaces, especially around the bed and the path to the bathroom, and to use night-lights. High-risk patients also need to know when and whom to call with specific foot problems. Patients with a puncture wound, ulcer, redness, or new-onset foot pain should call and see their primary care provider or podiatrist that day. Patients with callus and/or thick or ingrown nails should call a podiatrist and be seen within a few days.

Foot care educational materials for patients are available from NDEP in English and in Spanish at http://www.ndep.nih.gov/diabetes/pubs/Feet_broch_Eng.pdf (42).

To obtain free print copies of these patient education materials, the Feet Can Last a Lifetime health care provider kit, and other materials on diabetes prevention and control visit http://www.ndep.nih.gov or call 1-800-438-5383.

High and Low-Risk Foot Patient Education

The goal for low-risk patients is to keep them low risk:

- Control the ABCs.
- Tobacco cessation.

The goal for high-risk patients is to prevent foot ulcers:

- Self-management education:
- Stress the role of minor trauma.
- Clear walking spaces of potential hazards.
- Prompt (same day) care for injuries.
- Regular podiatry care.
- Use appropriate footwear.

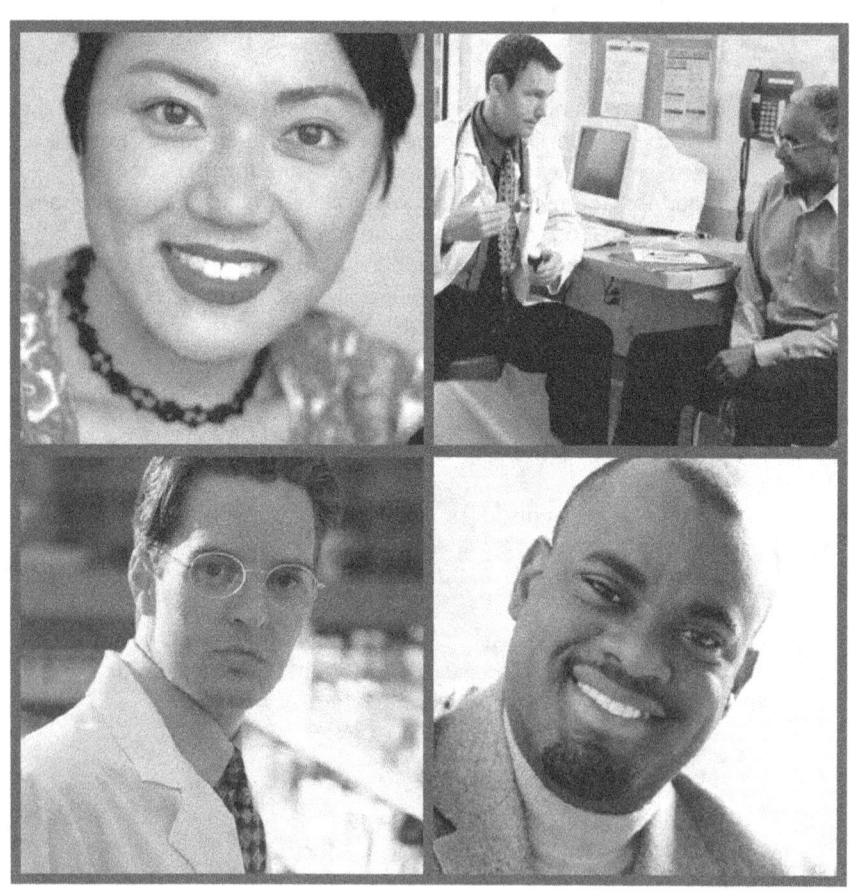

Section 6
Eye Health and Diabetes

Eye Health and Diabetes

Diabetes is the leading cause of new cases of blindness among adults aged 20 to 74 years. Diabetic retinopathy causes 12,000 to 24,000 new cases of blindness each year (43). People with diabetes can maintain optimal vision and healthy eyes by having an annual comprehensive vision examination, including a dilated eye examination, with early intervention if retinopathy is found.

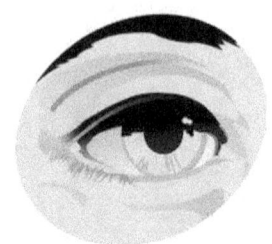

Diabetes-related Eye Conditions

People with diabetes are at 25 times greater risk for blindness (44). People with diabetes who smoke, have poor nutrition, and do not control their diabetes have an even greater risk of developing eye complications. Because many people with diabetes have slower healing time, eye injuries—even minor corneal scratches—should not be taken lightly.

Retinopathy

Diabetic retinopathy (DR) is a common complication of diabetes. Elevated blood sugar damages the retinal blood vessels, causing them to break down, leak, or become blocked. Over time, this causes retinal hemorrhage and impaired oxygen delivery to the retina that can lead to the growth of abnormal vessels. These new vessels are fragile and can break easily, causing permanent vision loss. One in 12 people with diabetes aged 40 years and older has vision-threatening diabetic retinopathy (45). Studies have shown that aspirin use (e.g., for CVD prophylaxis) is safe in persons with retinopathy and has no adverse effect on the development or progression of diabetic retinopathy (46, 47).

Poor glycemic control and longer duration of diabetes lead to increased rates of retinopathy in people with type 1 and type 2 diabetes. Diabetic retinopathy, however, is treatable, and one of the most preventable causes of vision loss and blindness. The risks of DR are reduced through disease management of blood sugar, blood pressure, and lipid control. Early diagnosis and proper treatment reduce the risk of vision loss; however, as many as 50% of patients are not getting their eyes examined or are diagnosed too late for treatment to be effective. Individuals with diabetes are also at an increased risk for glaucoma and cataracts.

Early detection and treatment can prevent or delay blindness due to diabetic retinopathy in 90% of people with diabetes. Good glycemic control has been shown to reduce or delay by 76% the development of retinopathy in people with diabetes (47). Intensive therapy reduces the first appearance of any retinopathy by 27%. Retinal laser photocoagulation surgery can reduce the risk of severe vision loss from the worst form of the disease, proliferative diabetic retinopathy (PDR), to 4% percent or less (48).

Optometrists and ophthalmologists can provide low-vision aids—from simple hand magnifiers to innovative optical devices—to help those who have experienced uncorrectable vision loss due to diabetic retinopathy. These eye care professionals can additionally provide or assure the provision of a full spectrum of care and services that may allow people with vision impairment and diabetes to maintain their independence and quality of life and help control their diabetes (e.g., to read instructions, take medication, continue with household tasks).

Other Common Eye Complications in Diabetes

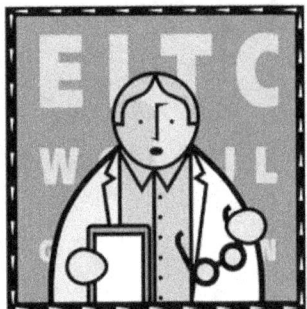

Cataracts are a clouding of the eye lens most often caused by aging. The lens is responsible for focusing the images onto the retina, and thus a clouding of the lens can result in diminished vision and increased sensitivity to glare. Over half of all Americans aged 65 years and older have cataracts (3).

Glaucoma is a progressive disease that damages the optic nerve. It is this nerve that carries the retinal image to the brain, so disruption of this transmission can cause irreversible blind spots or field loss, which over time can lead to total blindness. A view of the optic nerve during a dilated eye exam, combined with visual field testing, intraocular pressure testing (IOP), and other tests can often reveal damage at an early stage, thus providing opportunity for treatment. It is important to note that IOP should never be used as a sole diagnostic indicator. Among Americans aged 40 years or older, 2.2 million have glaucoma and another 1.1 million are unaware of having the disease (46). For this reason, glaucoma often is referred to as the "silent thief of sight." Glaucoma is twice as common among older black adults as among whites.

Double vision. People with diabetes may complain about sudden onset of double images. Because this can be due to damage to the nerves from the brain to the eye, it is important to see an optometrist or ophthalmologist immediately. This symptom can be misinterpreted by the patient or by a non-eye care provider unfamiliar with this ocular complication as a sign of a stroke or other neurological problem, prompting unnecessary diagnostic procedures such as radiological exams. Double vision (or diplopia) may instead be due to mononeuropathy—damage to a single nerve—usually cranial nerves III, IV, or VI. The sixth and third nerves are most frequently affected. Third-nerve palsies occur with pupillary sparing in 80% of cases. Most diabetic third-nerve palsies usually resolve spontaneously within 2 to 3 months and the symptom of double vision can often be controlled with the use of special lenses.

Vision fluctuation. Poor control of blood glucose levels can lead to a fluctuation in vision. These temporary visual fluctuations occur because of fluid imbalance in the crystalline lens. When the glucose level is elevated, the lens thickens, causing vision changes that may increase nearsightedness or farsightedness. When the glucose level returns to normal, the lens can shrink back to its normal state. For those who need glasses, if the glucose level is poorly controlled, the constant state of flux can make it difficult to determine the best lenses.

Comprehensive Dilated Eye Exam—
How Often and by Whom?

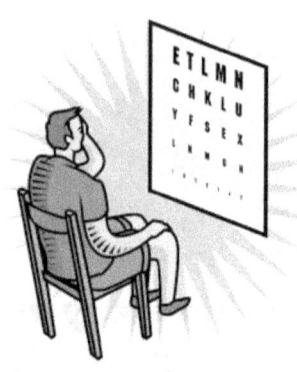

- Most people with diabetes should have a dilated eye examination by an optometrist or an ophthalmologist annually.

- If a person with diabetes has had a normal result for their eye exam, an eye care provider may suggest less frequent exams (every 2–3 years (30).

- Examinations will be needed more frequently if retinopathy exists or is progressing.

People with diabetes should have an exam by an eye specialist. A primary care medical professional (physician, nurse practitioner, or physician assistant) does not have the training, or often the equipment, to do a comprehensive diabetes eye exam.

Section 7

Oral Health and Diabetes

Oral Health and Diabetes

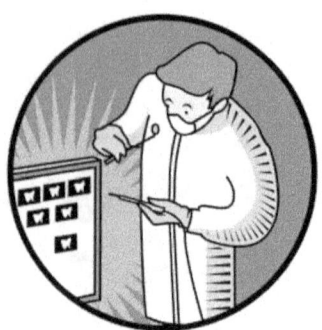

Changes in the Oral Cavity

Diabetes can lead to changes in the oral cavity. Of particular concern to dentists and dental hygienists are the effects of diabetes on the health of the gingiva (gums) and periodontal tissues (49). Poor glycemic control is associated with gingivitis and more severe periodontal diseases (50–52). Oral signs and symptoms of diabetes can also include a neurosensory disorder known as burning mouth syndrome, taste disorders, abnormal wound healing, and fungal infections (candidiasis). Individuals with diabetes may notice a fruity (acetone) breath, frequent xerostomia (dry mouth), or a change in saliva thickness. Dry mouth can also lead to a marked increase in dental decay. Oral findings in people with diabetes are associated with other systemic findings such as excessive loss of fluids through frequent urination, altered response to infection, altered connective tissue metabolism, neurosensory dysfunction, microvascular changes, medications causing dry mouth, and possible increased glucose concentration in saliva (53). Smoking often makes these problems worse. Unfortunately, caring for the mouth is often overlooked when trying to control other problems associated with diabetes. Good oral hygiene combined with good glycemic control can prevent many of these problems.

Periodontal Disease

People with diabetes are two to three times more likely than persons without diabetes to have destructive periodontal disease, such as periodontitis (54). Periodontal disease is a bacterially induced, chronic inflammatory disease that destroys the connective tissue and bone supporting the teeth and can lead to tooth loss. Periodontal disease is more prevalent, progresses more rapidly, and is often more severe in individuals with both type 1 and type 2 diabetes (55). Recent research suggests a two-way connection between diabetes and periodontal disease. Not only are people with diabetes more susceptible to periodontal disease, but the presence of periodontal disease may also make glycemic control more difficult (56-59). Proper care of the mouth that includes treatment of peridontal disease may help people with diabetes achieve better glycemic control.

Figure 6. U.S. Adults, Ages 45+, with Severe, "Active" Periodontitis* by Glycemic Control Status

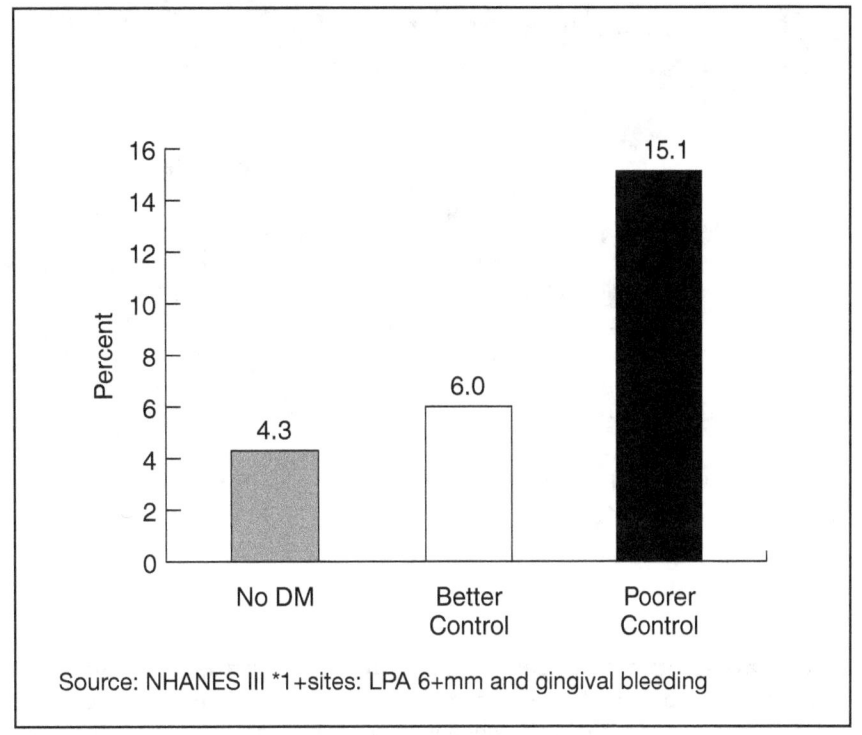

Source: NHANES III *1+sites: LPA 6+mm and gingival bleeding

Some studies have suggested a relationship between insulin resistance and inflammatory mediators. The inflamed periodontal tissue, which can be equivalent to an area as large as an adult palm, is highly vascular and may become ulcerated. This infection may introduce inflammatory mediators, as well as bacterial lipopolysaccharides and other toxins, into the systemic circulation. Some of the inflammatory mediators produced in periodontitis also stimulate the liver to produce acute-phase proteins, such as C-reactive protein (CRP), serum amyloid A, and fibrinogen. These proteins can be elevated in the peripheral blood of patients with periodontitis (60) and are associated with harmful effects on organs. Thus, periodontal inflammation potentially contributes to a systemic, chronic inflammatory state that also is a component of other inflammation-related diseases, including diabetes mellitus, cardiovascular diseases, and others. Treatment of periodontal disease decreases periodontal inflammation, and evidence is accumulating to support periodontal treatment contributing to improvement of glycemic control (61).

Recognize Oral Signs that may be Symptomatic for Diabetes:

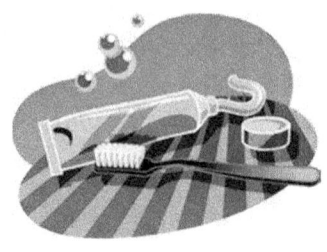

- Xerostomia
  - Dry mouth may also cause an increase in dental decay

- Periodontal (gum) disease
  - Red, swollen or bleeding gums
  - Gums pulling away from teeth
  - Abscesses (pus) between gums
  - Loose teeth or change in bite or tooth position

- Candidal infection (thrush)

- Persistent bad breath or bad taste, or fruity, acetone odor

Signs and symptoms of severe periodontal disease can include red, swollen, tender and bleeding gums; gums that have pulled away from the teeth; pus between the gums when they are compressed; persistent bad breath or bad taste in the mouth; permanent teeth that are loose or moving apart; any change in the way the teeth fit together when the patient bites; and any change in the fit of removable partial dentures. Most people with diabetes do not experience pain with periodontal disease, and many have periodontal disease and be asymptomatic. This highlights the importance of regular professional check-ups and care. Periodontal probing performed by a dentist or dental hygienist is a primary diagnostic assessment tool and can be used to measure response to treatment.

Section 8

Drug Therapy Management and Diabetes

Drug Therapy Management and Diabetes

Drug therapy management has traditionally been concerned with ensuring correct dosage, avoiding drug interactions, and educating patients about possible side effects. People identified as being at high risk for medication-related problems include those with chronic and multiple diseases, those who take multiple (five or more) medications, and those who see multiple health care providers. Because people with diabetes often fall into these categories, drug therapy management is especially important. It includes comprehensive reviews of medication and medical records, education of patients to improve compliance with medication regimens, and an assessment of individual response to therapy to ensure timely interventions and coordination and continuity of care.

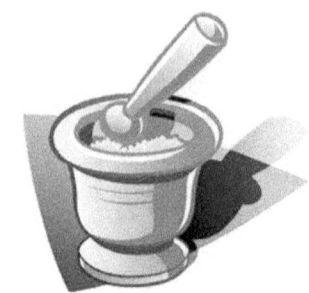

Drug-related Problems

Today's pharmaceuticals and advanced medical technologies provide many therapeutic options for treating diabetes and its comorbidities. If used inappropriately, however, they can cause serious illness, long-term disability, or even death. A study released in February 2001 shows that misuse of prescription drugs in the United States costs $177 billion annually in additional treatments, hospital care, and doctor visits, up from $76.5 billion in 1995. More important than the costs, however, the study estimates that 218,000 prescription drug-related deaths annually are due to misused prescription medications (62). The study identifies several categories of drug-related problems, including improper drug choice, underdosage, overdosage, adverse drug reactions, drug interactions, and undertreatment. Additional identified factors include untreated medical conditions and medication use with no indication (63, 64). More than 50% of those with chronic disorders do not take their medication properly. Over 60% of persons with diabetes do not adequately control their blood glucose. Of persons treated for high blood pressure and high cholesterol, 65% and 49%, respectively, are unable to reach target blood pressure and total cholesterol levels (65). To improve compliance and minimize these health care adversities, medication therapy regimens must be consistently and carefully monitored. Correct use of medication improves health and saves money for the health care system (66–68).

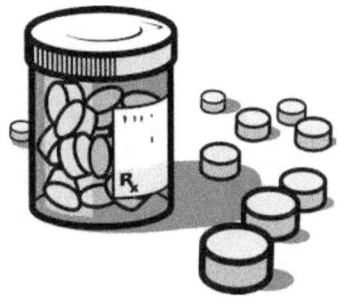

Strategies for Managing Drug Therapy

People with diabetes should establish a relationship with a pharmacist who can help monitor drug regimens, advise how to take medications properly, and provide other information to help them control their diabetes. Strategies include the following:

- **Use of medications.** Individualize drug regimens to determine the best time to take medications to reduce side effects and drug interactions. Offer behavior strategies, compliance aids, appropriate dosage forms, and a drug delivery system.

- **Self-treatment and over-the-counter medications.** Ask patients with diabetes if they are using nonprescription medications; vitamin, herbal, or nutritional supplements; or topical and skin-care products. Assess the severity and urgency of the person's complaint, the appropriateness for self-treatment, and any precautions and contraindications. Recommend self-treatment, follow-up, and/or referral to another health care professional, as appropriate.

One study reported that over 57% of people with diabetes use complemetary and alternative therapies (69).

- **Selecting and using a blood glucose meter.** Help the patient choose an appropriate blood glucose meter and provide training on how to use it. Educate the person about the results, actions to take, and when to seek help. Self-monitoring blood glucose (SMBG) is an important way to assess the effectiveness of therapy.

- **Cost control.** Advise on ways to decrease costs of medications and supplies by providing information on private insurance plans, prescription drug programs, Medicare and Medicaid, the role of generic medications, and possible coverage for referrals to other health care providers.

Section 9

Coordination of Care

Coordination of Care

Coordination of care presents many challenges when delivered by multiple providers in a variety of settings. Changes in drug therapy may occur when patients see specialty providers or during acute illness or hospitalization. When a case includes multiple disease states and multiple drugs, along with OTC drugs, herbal products, and other supplements, diligent case management is required to ensure continuity of care that is well coordinated (69).

As an extension of the dispensing role of pharmacists, central medication review and drug therapy management (including nonprescription products) can ensure that a current drug therapy plan is appropriately implemented. In one study, collaborative drug therapy management (CDTM), provided by pharmacists in collaboration with other health care providers, resulted in identification of problems in 65% of patients' drug regimens (70). In other studies, CDTM resulted in decreased morbidity and mortality, as well as decreased costs attributable to fewer unscheduled physician visits, urgent care visits, emergency room visits, and hospital days (71–73).

With coordinated care, all members of the health care team, including the patient, benefit from having a primary resource to deliver intended drug therapy, information, and monitoring for effectiveness and adverse effects. This coordination will help ensure adherence to the intended treatment plan and identify drug and disease management problems in a timely manner.

Coordination of Care:

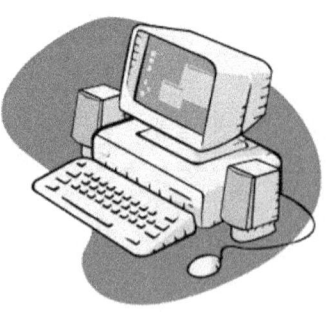

- Engage clinic leadership in establishing diabetes quality care in the strategic plan.

- Support a designated diabetes coordinator and diabetes team.

- Provide self-management education services according to the NDEP and ADA standards.

- System redesign:

    -Use registries and tracking systems for appointments.

    -Prescreen charts to prepare for the office visit.

    -Case management through a care coordinator.

- Decision support such as flow sheets and electronic health record automated prompts.

- Establish links to community resources.

Section 10

Pre-diabetes and Primary Prevention

Pre-diabetes and Primary Prevention

An estimated 54 million Americans aged 40 to 74 years (40.1% of the U.S. population in this age group) have pre-diabetes, a condition that puts them at high risk for developing type 2 diabetes. Without intervention, people with pre-diabetes will progress to type 2 diabetes at a rate of 10% per year. Pre-diabetes also increases the risk of heart disease and stroke (3).

Pre-diabetes is a condition in which blood glucose levels are higher than normal but not in the diabetes range. Pre-diabetes is defined as impaired fasting glucose (IFG) of 100 to 125 mg/dl or impaired glucose tolerance (IGT) diagnosed by a post 75-gram glucose challenge (oral glucose tolerance test or OGTT) of >140 to <200 mg/dl or both IFG and IGT. (See appendix B for more information on blood glucose testing.) The Am I at Risk for Type 2 Diabetes? brochure, produced by the National Institute of Diabetes and Digestive and Kidney Diseases (NIDDK), can help patients and providers assess individual risk for Pre-diabetes.

Primary Prevention

Primary prevention refers to preventing diabetes from occurring. Secondary prevention refers to preventing complications in those who already have diabetes (e.g., prevention of neuropathy) and tertiary prevention refers to prevention of worsening complications (e.g., amputation resulting from injury to a neuropathic foot) or death.

The burden of diabetes is high. On average, more than 4,100 people are diagnosed with diabetes every day. On average, 55 go blind, 120 experience kidney failure, and 230 have a limb amputated every day. The rate of prevalence increase is high. In the past 25 years, the number of Americans with diabetes has more than tripled (from 5.8 million to 20.8 million), and future projections are high.

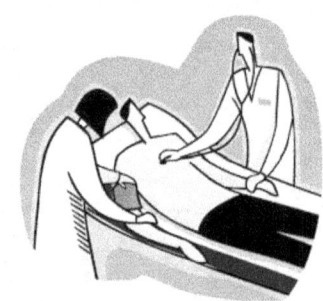

It is estimated that of persons born in America in 2002, 1 in 3 will develop diabetes in his or her lifetime. For Hispanic/Latino women, the statistic is 1 in 2...unless something changes.

Trend is not Destiny

Type 2 diabetes can be prevented or delayed. A major clinical trial—the Diabetes Prevention Program (DPP) study—provided scientific evidence that the onset of diabetes could be prevented or delayed in people at high risk. In the DPP, adults with Pre-diabetes reduced their risk of developing diabetes during the course of the study by 58% through such lifestyle changes as:

* Reduced fat and calorie intake.
* Increased physical activity of at least 150 minutes/week (e.g., brisk walking 30 minutes a day, 5 days/week).
* Loss of more than 5% to 7% of body weight.

Table 6.

Test	Value	Diagnosis
FPG*	100–125 mg/dL	IFG (pre-diabetes)
FPG	>125 mg/dL	Diabetes
OGTT**	2-hour value 140–199 mg/dL	IGT (pre-diabetes)
OGTT	2-hour value >200mg/dL	Diabetes

*FPG = fasting plasma glucose
**OGTT = oral glucose tolerance test, blood glucose measured 2 hours after 75gm glucose load

These lifestyle changes were effective in preventing or delaying diabetes in all ages and all ethnic groups in the DPP. Among people aged 60 years and older, progression to type 2 diabetes was reduced by 71%. The DPP showed that moderate changes resulting in modest weight loss can make a difference (9).

DPP participants have been enrolled in a continuation study and follow-up data will be forthcoming. Further information on pre-diabetes, testing recommendations, and information on the NDEP's Small Steps. Big Rewards. Prevent Type 2 Diabetes. campaign and tools can be found on the NDEP Web site at http://ndep.nih.gov/campaigns/SmallSteps/SmallSteps_index.htm.

The Role of PPOD Providers in Primary Prevention

All health care providers can play a role in diabetes primary prevention and diabetes control. As a pharmacist, podiatrist, optometrist, dentist, or dental hygienist, you can make a difference in primary prevention:

- You know your patients.
- Your patients trust you.
- A few words from you can go a long way.
- You can determine with just a few questions who is at high risk for diabetes (see risk factor list below).

Do Your Patients Have any of the Following Risk Factors?

- Family history of type 2 diabetes.
- Overweight or obesity.
- High blood pressure or cholesterol.
- African American, American Indian/Alaska Native, Asian American, Hispanic/Latino, Native Hawaiian/Pacific Islander ethnicity.
- Pre-diabetes.
- Age of more than 45 years.
- History of gestational diabetes (GDM).

Gestational Diabetes Mellitus (GDM)

It is estimated that women who have had GDM have a 20% to 50% likelihood of developing type 2 diabetes in the 5 to 10 years following pregnancy. Without intervention, progression from Pre-diabetes to type 2 diabetes occurs at a rate of approximately 10% per year. With NDEP resources and self-management support for behavior change, diabetes can be prevented or delayed.

A Few Words Can Go a Long Way

You don't need to do it all—resources are available to help. Your patients will appreciate that you care about their overall health

Ask: "Has anyone ever told you that you are at risk for diabetes?"
Advise: "You can take action to prevent or delay type 2 diabetes."
Assist: Give your patients resources to help them make healthy changes:
  • Refer to a primary care provider.
  • Use the free primary prevention materials available from the National

Diabetes Education Program (NDEP)—call 1-800-438-5383, visit www.ndep.nih.gov or use the order form in the Appendix.

Primary Prevention Hypothetical Cases

  • A 30-year-old woman at a routine dental hygienist appointment shares that fact that she recently delivered a nine-pound baby after a pregnancy complicated by GDM. She exclaims "Thank goodness that's all over!" The dental hygienist tells her of the high lifelong risk of developing type 2 diabetes in women who have had GDM. The patient learns about the free NDEP materials available to help her lose weight and prevent or delay the onset of type 2 diabetes.

  • A 45-year-old African American woman brings her mother in for her annual comprehensive diabetes eye exam. The eye care provider asks if she ever considered that she, too, might be at risk for developing diabetes. The woman is surprised. "Me? I just never thought much about it. I've always been focused on Mama." The eye care provider gives the woman the Am I At Risk? brochure, NDEP's toll-free number and Web site URL, and suggests she make a follow-up appointment with her own primary care provider.

  • A 50-year-old man accompanied by his overweight teenage son asks the pharmacist about weight loss pills. The pharmacist asks to talk to both father and son together. The teen seems embarrassed and unconvinced. He says "What am I supposed to eat when the guys are all eating cheeseburgers and fries after school?!" The pharmacist agrees that changing eating habits is hard, but not impossible. Smaller portions, or choosing a plain hamburger instead of the oversized one with cheese, can make a difference. He suggests the family take a look at NDEP's Web site for tip sheets on healthy eating and physical activity, and that they talk to a dietitian. Dad agrees to play basketball with his son a couple of nights a week—good exercise for both of them.

  • A 70-year-old man consults a podiatrist because of painful corns on his feet. He says "I don't walk anymore because of these corns, but I guess that doesn't matter—I'm too old to be walking much now." The podiatrist emphasizes the many benefits of regular physical activity such as walking, including diabetes prevention. He explains that 1 in 5 people over age 60 have diabetes, but that the disease can be prevented or delayed. He shares the NDEP "It's Not Too Late to Prevent Diabetes" tip sheet with the man and points out NDEP's toll-free number and URL. He says, "After we get these corns fixed up, I want to see you out there walking!"

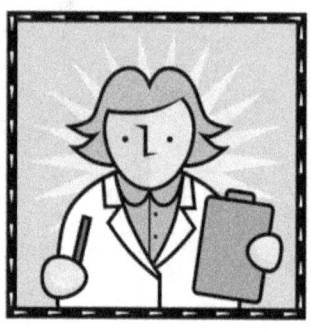

Always advise patients to check with their primary care provider before beginning an exercise or physical activity program.

Appendices

Appendix A

Set Up a Referral System

Integrated, multidisciplinary team care is key to successful diabetes management, and coordination of care can be facilitated by setting up a system of referrals for routine preventive care as well as for urgent needs.

Create a mechanism for preventive care and urgent referrals; don't just tell the person with a potentially serious problem to consult a health specialist right away. Contact primary care and specialty providers to discuss with them criteria and ensure that procedures are in place for seeing a person who is referred for preventive care or an urgent basis.

Make a list of providers, case managers, phone numbers, and other contact information; keep it handy for quick reference. Consider giving individuals handouts with referral information, or calling clinics directly for urgent referrals.

Check the NDEP health care providers' Web site, http://www.betterdiabetescare.nih.gov, for tools to help set up a referral system.

Appendix B

Blood Glucose Testing

Diagnosis is based on plasma glucose levels obtained from a venous sample (74). Information on diagnostic criteria, relative merits of different screening tests, and an algorithm for evaluating people at risk can be found at http://ndep.nih.gov/ddi/#HC. Blood glucose testing can be performed using different methods for different purposes.

Screening refers to testing asymptomatic individuals at high risk for diabetes via venous sample (preferred) or a capillary sample to determine if follow-up diagnostic testing is indicated (75).

Blood glucose testing to monitor glycemic status by patients and health care providers is considered a cornerstone of diabetes care. Results of monitoring are used to assess the efficacy of therapy and guide adjustments in medical nutrition therapy (MNT), exercise, and medications to achieve the best possible glucose control (76).

Blood glucose testing by people with diabetes—self-monitoring of blood glucose (SMBG)—is recommended for all people with type 1 diabetes. For most such patients, SMBG three or more times a day is recommended. For people with type 2 diabetes, the frequency of testing should be sufficient to facilitate reaching glucose goals. The frequency of testing should be increased with therapy modification (77).

Because the accuracy of SMBG depends on both the instrument and the user, the technique should be evaluated by a health care provider initially and then periodically (78).

Requirements for Laboratory Testing

All health care providers who perform finger sticks or other laboratory testing must be registered with the Centers for Medicare & Medicaid Services (CMS) under the Clinical Laboratory Improvement Amendment (CLIA), which established quality standards to ensure the accuracy, reliability, and timeliness of patient test results regardless of where the test is performed. Three categories of tests and certification have been established, depending on the complexity of the test method. CLIA has established compliance regulations for each level of testing that require quality control and documentation procedures (79).

Certain states have established additional requirements for various sites or health care providers. For specific additional requirements, health care providers should contact their state agency (see http://www.cms.hhs.gov/clia for contact information). Compliance with the Occupational Safety and Health Administration's regulations for bloodborne pathogens must also be documented and maintained.

Appendix C

Multidisciplinary Care in Action

People with diabetes may present with a complaint best treated with multidisciplinary care. Common symptoms or concerns and possible presentation and management scenarios are given below as examples.

Foot and Skin Care

- Dry skin.
- Wounds, fungal and bacterial infections, ulcers.
- Pain, numbness, tingling of extremities.
- Corns, calluses, bunions, ingrown toenails.

Example:

A person requests a foot soak from the pharmacist for an ingrown toenail. Assessment reveals that he or she has diabetes and for 3 weeks has had a severely inflamed ingrown toenail that has not responded to topical antibiotic ointment. The pharmacist discusses with the person the relationship between diabetes and its complications, as well as the need to seek immediate attention from a podiatrist or primary care physician. The pharmacist also emphasizes that people with diabetes should NOT soak their feet. Soaking dries the skin and can cause more skin and foot complications.

Eye Health

- Dry itchy eyes.
- Blurred vision, poor vision (seeking reading glasses).
- Eye pain.
- Conjunctivitis.
- Other eye problems such as partial vision, hemorrhages, floaters, "spots," foreign objects, contact lens problems.

Example:

A 45-year-old woman tells her podiatrist that she can't check her feet because she "just can't see as well" as she used to. She was recently diagnosed with diabetes. She assumed that she needed reading glasses, but has not had an eye exam because she never had poor vision before. The podiatrist recognizes that the patient's blurred vision could be a sign of poor glucose control or eye pathology, and explains to her the relationship between diabetes and vision problems, both transient and long term. The podiatrist then refers the patient to an optometrist or an ophthalmologist for a comprehensive eye examination, including pupil dilation, and to a primary care provider for follow-up.

Oral Health

- Sore, red, inflamed, bleeding gums.
- Toothache, pain, infections.
- Dry mouth.
- Candida infections.
- Denture pain.
- Cold sores, canker sores.

Example:

A person with diabetes asks the pharmacist for a product to use as a mouth rinse for irritated gums. Assessment reveals that the person has poorly controlled diabetes and symptoms consistent with oral candida infection. The pharmacist briefly explains the relationship between diabetes and oral health, and refers the patient to a dentist for treatment. Follow-up care for diabetes with a primary care provider is also arranged.

Medication Management

- Multiple medications.
- Varying instructions on how to take medications.
- Drug-drug interactions.
- Over-the-counter treatments, herbals, home remedies.
- Symptoms attributed to medication side effects.

Example:

A dental hygienist asks if a patient's medications have changed since the last visit and discovers the patient is confused about how to take a newly prescribed medicine. The patient asks if "twice a day" means with breakfast and dinner, morning and bedtime, or at precise times such as 8 a.m. and 8 p.m. He further asks if the medication may be taken at the same time as other medications, because he takes several other medications for blood pressure and cholesterol as well as glucose control. He states: "It's hard to find time to take all these medicines in one day!" The dental hygienist reinforces the importance of taking the medicine as directed, and suggests consulting with the provider who prescribed the medicines and with the pharmacist to ask these questions. The pharmacist may be more immediately accessible, can provide counseling on potential drug interactions, and can work with patients who are on complicated medicine regimens to work out an individualized schedule.

Appendix D

Medication Supplement and Patient Education Poster

Working Together to Manage Diabetes has two companion pieces: a *Working Together Medications Supplement* and patient education poster (available in English and Spanish).

The *Working Together Medications Supplement* is a quick reference guide to medications commonly used by people who have diabetes, and is intended to help providers understand these medications. For complete prescribing information, please consult the package inserts or the *Physicians' Desk Reference*.

PPOD providers and others not only can use the *Working Together Medications Supplement* to reinforce patient education messages about medication use, but also to coordinate team care. For example:

- Types of insulin and timing of their administration may help the PPOD provider schedule a procedure at an appropriate time.
- Awareness of common medication-related symptoms can help a non-primary care provider recognize a potential problem and make a referral.
- Adverse interaction of medications prescribed by multiple providers can be reduced.
- Inadvertent over and underdosing can be lessened if the entire health care team is aware of medication names (both generic and trade names), strengths, and dosing frequency.
- Every patient interaction is an opportunity to reinforce correct use of medication and to refer as needed to the primary care clinician and pharmacist for individualized drug therapy counseling.

The *Working Together to Manage Diabetes* patient education poster focuses on the steps a person with diabetes can take to team up with their PPOD providers for foot, eye, and oral health care and medication management. The poster emphasizes proactive "I will" statements and shows photos of PPOD providers interacting with patients. The poster can be hung in a waiting room, the public area of a pharmacy or community hall, or used as a prompt on key messages in one-on-one patient counseling.

The *Working Together Medications Supplement* and patient education posters are available for downloading from www.ndep.nih.gov and are copyright-free. Single free hard copies can be ordered via the National Diabetes Education Program Web site or by calling 1-800-438-5383.

Additional Resources

American Academy of Ophthalmology

http://www.aao.org/

The American Academy of Ophthalmology has more than 27,000 members worldwide. Academy members are doctors of medicine or osteopathy who specialize in the eyes and vision. The majority are practicing physicians who provide the full spectrum of eye care, from prescribing glasses and contact lenses, to the medical and surgical treatment of a wide variety of eye conditions. In addition, many are subspecialists with special training who focus their practices in specific areas of ophthalmology such as glaucoma, cataract, or pediatric ophthalmology.

American Academy of Optometry

http://www.aaopt.org

Founded in 1922, the goal of the American Academy of Optometry is to maintain and enhance excellence in optometric practice by fostering research and the dissemination of knowledge in both basic and applied vision science.

American Academy of Periodontology

http://www.perio.org

The mission of the American Academy of Periodontology is to advance the periodontal health of the public and to represent and serve the Academy's members. It provides clinical and scientific publications as well as consumer information.

American Association of Clinical Endocrinologists

http://www.aace.com

The American Association of Clinical Endocrinologists is a professional medical organization devoted to the enhancement of the practice of clinical endocrinology. Its members are physicians with special education, training, and interest in the practice of clinical endocrinology.

American Association of Diabetes Educators

800-TEAM-UP4

http://www.aadenet.org

The American Association of Diabetes Educators is a multidisciplinary organization representing health care professionals who provide diabetes education and care. It provides continuing education and products for health care professionals in all settings.

American College of Clinical Pharmacy

http://www.accp.com

The American College of Clinical Pharmacy provides leadership, education, advocacy, and resources to enable clinical pharmacists to achieve excellence in practice and research. It provides research forums, continuing education, publications, and a practice and research network.

American Dental Association

http://www.ada.org

The American Dental Association is the professional association of dentists committed to the public's oral health, as well as ethics, science, and professional advancement. It provides continuing education and a monthly journal for dentists, in addition to consumer education on oral health topics.

American Dental Hygienists Association

800-243-ADHA

http://www.adha.org/

The American Dental Hygienists Association is the largest professional organization representing the interests of dental hygienists. It provides continuing education through its Institute for Oral Health, as well as information on oral health topics, careers in dental hygiene, and professional issues.

American Diabetes Association

800-342-2383

http://www.diabetes.org

The American Diabetes Association funds research; publishes scientific findings; provides information and other services to people with diabetes, their families, health care professionals, and the public; and advocates for scientific research and the rights of people with diabetes.

American Dietetic Association

800-366-1655

http://www.eatright.org

The American Dietetic Association is the nation's largest organization of food and nutrition professionals. Its mission is to promote optimal nutrition and well-being for all people by advocating for its members.

American Optometric Association

http://www.aoa.org

The mission of the American Optometric Association is to influence the future of eye care by ensuring the welfare of the public and promoting the profession of optometry. Its objectives are centered on improving the quality and availability of eye and vision care.

American Pharmacists Association

http://www.aphanet.org

The American Pharmacists Association is the largest national professional society of pharmacists. It is a leader in providing professional information and in advocating for the improved health of the American public through the provision of comprehensive pharmaceutical care.

American Podiatric Medical Association

http://www.apma.org

The American Podiatric Medical Association represents approximately 80% of the nation's podiatrists and has more than 20 affiliated and related societies. Its mission is to increase awareness among other health professionals and the public concerning the importance of foot health.

American Public Health Association

http://www.apha.org

The American Public Health Association is the oldest and largest organization of public health professionals in the world, representing more than 50,000 members from over 50 occupations of public health. The Association brings together researchers, health service providers, administrators, teachers, and other health workers in a unique, multidisciplinary environment of professional exchange, study, and action.

American Society of Health-System Pharmacists

http://www.ashp.org

The American Society of Health-System Pharmacists represents pharmacists who practice in hospitals and other components of health care systems. It provides extensive publishing, education, and accreditation programs designed to help members improve their delivery of pharmaceutical care.

HRSA Health Disparities Collaboratives

http://www.healthdisparities.net

The Health Disparities Collaboratives is a program that includes the Bureau of Primary Health Care, Institute for Healthcare Improvement, National Association of Community Health Centers, Inc., and other strategic partners, to generate and document improved health outcomes for underserved populations; transform clinical practice through models of care, improvement, and learning; develop infrastructure, expertise, and multidisciplinary leadership to support and drive improved health status; and build strategic partnerships.

Centers for Disease Control and Prevention Division of Diabetes Translation

877-232-3422

http://www.cdc.gov/diabetes

CDC's Division of Diabetes Translation aims to reduce the nation's burden of diabetes by strengthening public health surveillance systems, conducting applied transnational research, developing state-based diabetes control programs, implementing the National Diabetes Education Program (NDEP), and providing public information.

Centers for Medicare & Medicaid Services

410-786-3000

http://www.cms.gov

The Centers for Medicare & Medicaid Services, formerly known as the Health Care Financing Administration, is the federal agency responsible for administering Medicare, Medicaid, the State Children's Health Insurance Program, and several other health-related programs.

Indian Health Services Diabetes Program

http://www.ihs.gov/MedicalPrograms/Diabetes/index.asp

The Indian Health Service provides health care to 1.6 million Native Americans and Alaska Indians from more than 550 federally recognized tribes across the nation. Diabetes is a major concern among the treatment population and the Division of Diabetes Treatment and Prevention has made numerous tools and information available on their Web site to assist with this epidemic, including best practices for eye care, foot care, oral health, and pharmaceutical care.

National Association of Chain Drug Stores

http://www.nacds.org

The National Association of Chain Drug Stores provides a wide range of services to meet the needs of the chain drug industry, including publications for members and information for consumers.

National Community Pharmacists Association

http://www.ncpanet.org

The National Community Pharmacists Association represents the nation's community pharmacists, including the owners of nearly 24,000 independent pharmacies that generate more than $67 billion in annual sales and dispense nearly half of all retail prescriptions. The Association is committed to high-quality pharmacist care and to promoting the health and well being of the public.

National Diabetes Education Program

http://www.ndep.nih.gov

http://www.cdc.gov/diabetes/ndep

http://www.diabetesatwork.org

http://www.betterdiabetescare.nih.gov

The National Diabetes Education Program brings together public and private partners to improve treatment and outcomes for people with diabetes, promote early diagnosis, and prevent the onset of type 2 diabetes. It promotes awareness and education activities and quality care. The Web site provides tools for educating health care providers and patients.

National Diabetes Information Clearinghouse

800-860-8747

http://diabetes.niddk.nih.gov

The NIDDK's National Diabetes Information Clearinghouse is an information and referral service designed to increase knowledge about diabetes among patients and their families, health care professionals, and the public.

National Eye Institute

301-496-5248

http://www.nei.nih.gov

The National Eye Institute conducts and supports research to help prevent and treat eye diseases and other disorders of vision, including diabetic retinopathy. It also develops public and professional education programs, including the National Eye Health Education Program, a partnership of more than 65 organizations concerned with eye health.

National Heart, Lung, and Blood Institute

301-592-8573

http://www.nhlbi.nih.gov

The National Heart, Lung, and Blood Institute provides leadership for a national program in diseases of the heart, blood vessels, lungs, and blood; blood resources; and sleep disorders. It supports research, develops and evaluates interventions, and conducts educational activities with an emphasis on prevention.

National Institute of Dental and Craniofacial Research

http://www.nidcr.nih.gov

The National Institute of Dental and Craniofacial Research (NIDCR) conducts and supports research and the training of researchers to promote the oral, dental, and craniofacial health of the American people, prevent oral diseases and conditions, and develop new diagnostics and therapeutics. Two useful publications developed for consumers are *Diabetes: Dental Tips* and *Prevent Diabetes Problems: Keep Your Teeth and Gums Healthy*.

National Institute of Diabetes and Digestive and Kidney Diseases

http://www.niddk.nih.gov

The National Institute of Diabetes and Digestive and Kidney Diseases (NIDDK) conducts and supports basic and clinical research on the treatment and prevention of diabetes and other serious diseases affecting metabolism and the endocrine system, digestion and nutrition, the kidneys and urinary tract, and the blood and blood-forming organs.

National Optometric Association

http://www.natoptassoc.org

The National Optometric Association promotes the recruitment of minority students for schools and colleges of optometry and their placement into appropriate practice settings upon graduation. It also works to enhance the delivery of eye and vision care services in communities with little or no eye care presence.

Selected Publications for Health Care Providers and Patients

(This list represents only a sample of materials available—please consult the Web sites indicated.)

Available from the Centers for Disease Control and Prevention (CDC)
http://www.cdc.gov/diabetes/pubs/tcyd/index.htm :

- Take Charge of Your Diabetes

Available from the National Diabetes Education Program (NDEP)
(See order form at end of appendices.)
http://www.ndep.nih.gov :

- Your GAMEPLAN for Preventing Type 2 Diabetes: Health Care Providers' Toolkit
- Your GAMEPLAN for Preventing Type 2 Diabetes: Information for Patients
- Team Care: Comprehensive Lifetime Management for Diabetes
- Feet Can Last a Lifetime: A Health Care Provider's Guide to Preventing Diabetes Foot Problems
- Diabetes Numbers At-a-Glance (card for health care providers)
- Be Smart About Your Heart
- 7 Principles for Controlling Your Diabetes
- If You Have Diabetes, Know Your Blood Sugar Numbers
- Control Your Diabetes. For Life. Tips for Feeling Better and Staying Healthy
- Asian language patient materials
- Spanish patient materials

References

1. Centers for Disease Control and Prevention. *National Diabetes Fact Sheet: General Information and National Estimates on Diabetes in the United States, 2005.* Atlanta, GA: U.S. Department of Health and Human Services, Centers for Disease Control and Prevention; 2005. Accessed 10/16/06 at: http://www.cdc.gov/diabetes/pubs/factsheet05.htm.

2. Hogan P, Dall T, Nikolov P. Economic costs of diabetes in the U.S. in 2002. *Diabetes Care.* 2003;26:917–32. [PMID: 12610059].[Abstract/Free Full Text]

3. Centers for Disease Control and Prevention. *National diabetes fact sheet: General information and national estimates on diabetes in the United States, 2005.* Atlanta, GA: U.S. Department of Health and Human Services, Centers for Disease Control and Prevention, 2005. Accessed 09/18/06 at: http://www.cdc.gov/diabetes/pubs/pdf/ndfs_2005.pdf.

4. Honeycutt AA, Boyle JP, Broglio KR, Thompson TJ, Hoerger TJ, Geiss LS, et al. A dynamic Markov model for forecasting diabetes prevalence in the United States through 2050. *Health Care Manag Sci.* 2003;6:155–64. [PMID: 12943151].[Medline]

5. Narayan KM, Boyle JP, Thompson TJ, Sorensen SW, Williamson DF. Lifetime risk for diabetes mellitus in the United States. *JAMA.* 2003;290:1884–90. [PMID: 14532317].[Abstract/Free Full Text]

6. Mokdad AH, Ford ES, Bowman BA, Nelson DE, Engelgaw MM. et al. Diabetes trends in the U.S. 1990–1998. *Diabetes Care* 2000;23:1278–1283.

7. Mokdad AH, Serdula MK, Dietz WH, Bowman BA, Marks JS, et al. The Spread of the obesity epidemic in the United States, 1991–1998. *JAMA* 1999; 282:1519–1522.

8. Mokdad AH, Bowman BA, Ford ES, Vinicor F, Marks JS, Koplan JP. The Continuing Epidemics of Obesity and Diabetes in the United States. *JAMA,* 2001; 286: 1195–1200.

9. Knowler WC, Barrett-Connor E, Fowler SE, Hamman RF, Lachin JM, Walker EA, et al. Reduction in the incidence of type 2 diabetes with lifestyle intervention or metformin. *N Engl J Med.* 2002;346:393–403. [Abstract/Free Full Text]

10. The effect of intensive treatment of diabetes on the development and progression of long-term complications in insulin-dependent diabetes mellitus. The Diabetes Control and Complications Trial Research Group. *N Engl J Med.* 1993;329:977–86. [PMID: 8366922].[Abstract/Free Full Text]

11. Intensive blood-glucose control with sulphonylureas or insulin compared with conventional treatment and risk of complications in patients with type 2 diabetes (UKPDS 33). UK Prospective Diabetes Study (UKPDS) Group. *Lancet.* 1998;352:837–53. [PMID: 9742976].[Medline]

12. Tight blood pressure control and risk of macrovascular and microvascular complications in type 2 diabetes: UKPDS 38. UK Prospective Diabetes Study Group. *BMJ.* 1998;317:703–13. [PMID: 9732337].[Abstract/Free Full Text]

13. Goldberg RB, Mellies MJ, Sacks FM, Moyé LA, Howard BV, Howard WJ, et al. Cardiovascular events and their reduction with pravastatin in diabetic and glucose-intolerant myocardial infarction survivors with average cholesterol levels: Subgroup analyses in the cholesterol and recurrent events (CARE) trial. The Care Investigators. *Circulation.* 1998;98:2513–9. [PMID: 9843456].[Abstract/Free Full Text]

14. Effects of ramipril on cardiovascular and microvascular outcomes in people with diabetes mellitus: Results of the HOPE study and MICRO-HOPE substudy. Heart Outcomes Prevention Evaluation Study Investigators. *Lancet.* 2000;355:253–9. [PMID: 10675071] [Medline]

15. Early photocoagulation for diabetic retinopathy. ETDRS report number 9. Early Treatment Diabetic Retinopathy Study Research Group. *Ophthalmology.* 1991;98:766–85. [PMID: 2062512] [Medline]

16. Litzelman DK, Slemenda CW, Langefeld CD, Hays LM, Welch MA, Bild DE, et al. Reduction of lower extremity clinical abnormalities in patients with non-insulin-dependent diabetes mellitus. A randomized, controlled trial. *Ann Intern Med.* 1993;119:36–41. [PMID: 8498761] [Abstract/Free Full Text]

17. Lifetime benefits and costs of intensive therapy as practiced in the diabetes control and complications trial. The Diabetes Control and Complications Trial Research Group. *JAMA.* 1996;276:1409–15. [PMID: 8892716] [Abstract]

18. Cost effectiveness analysis of improved blood pressure control in hypertensive patients with type 2 diabetes: UKPDS 40. UK Prospective Diabetes Study Group. *BMJ.* 1998;317:720–6. [PMID: 9732339] [Abstract/Free Full Text]

19. Schwartz JS, Boccuzzi SJ, Glick H, Cook JR, Pederson TR, Kjekshus J. Cost-effectiveness of LDL-C reduction in diabetic CHD patients: Implications from the Scandinavian Simvastatin Survival Study (4S). *Circulation.* 1997;96(suppl 1):1504–5. [Abstract]

20. Javitt JC, Aiello LP, Chiang Y, Ferris FL 3rd, Canner JK, Greenfield S. Preventive eye care in people with diabetes is cost-saving to the federal government. Implications for health-care reform. *Diabetes Care.* 1994;17:909–17. [PMID: 7956643].[Abstract]

21. Siegel JE, Krolewski AS, Warram JH, Weinstein MC. Cost-effectiveness of screening and early treatment of nephropathy in patients with insulin-dependent diabetes mellitus. *J Am Soc Nephrol.* 1992;3:S111-9. [PMID: 1457753].[Abstract]

22. Saaddine JB, Engelgau MM, Beckles GL, Gregg EW, Thompson TJ, Narayan KM. A diabetes report card for the United States: Quality of care in the 1990s. *Ann Intern Med.* 2002;136:565–74. [PMID: 11955024].[Abstract/Free Full Text]

23. Beckles GL, Engelgau MM, Narayan KM, Herman WH, Aubert RE, Williamson DF. Population-based assessment of the level of care among adults with diabetes in the U.S. *Diabetes Care.* 1998;21:1432–8. [PMID: 9727887].[Abstract]

24. Engelgau MM, Geiss LS, Manninen DL, Orians CE, Wagner EH, Friedman NM, et al. Use of services by diabetes patients in managed care organizations. Development of a diabetes surveillance system. CDC Diabetes in Managed Care Work Group. *Diabetes Care.* 1998;21:2062–8. [PMID: 9839095].[Abstract]

25. Kenny SJ, Smith PJ, Goldschmid MG, Newman JM, Herman WH. Survey of physician practice behaviors related to diabetes mellitus in the U.S. Physician adherence to consensus recommendations. *Diabetes Care.* 1993;16:1507–10. [PMID: 8299440].[Abstract]

26. Ohkubo Y, et al. Diabetes Res Clin Pract. 1995; 28:103–117.

27. American Diabetes Association Standards of Medical Care. *Diabetes Care* 2006; 29 (Suppl.1):S4–S42.

28. National Diabetes Education Program. *Team Care: Comprehensive Lifetime Management for Diabetes* (NDEP–37). Accessed 4/06/07 at http://ndep.nih.gov/diabetes/pubs/TeamCare.pdf.

29. Bodenheimer T, Lorig K, Holman H, Grumbach K. Patient self-management of chronic disease in primary care. *JAMA.*2002;288(19):2469–75.

30. American Diabetes Association Position Statement on Diabetic Retinopathy. *Diabetes Care.* 2004;27:Suppl 1: S84–S87.

31. Hospital discharge rates for non-traumatic lower extremity amputation by diabetes status—United States, 1997. *MMWR* 2001;50(43):954–8.

32. History of foot ulcer among persons with diabetes—United States, 2000–2002. *MMWR* 2003;52(45):1098–1102.

33. Armstrong DG, Lavery LA, Harkless LB. Validation of a diabetic wound classification system. The contribution of depth, infection, and ischemia to risk of amputation. *Diabetes Care.* 1998;21(5):855–9.

34. History of foot ulcer, op. cit.

35. Litzelman DK, Marriott DJ, Vinicor F. Independent physiological predictors of foot lesions in patients with NIDDM. *Diabetes Care.* 1997;20(8):1273–8.

36. American Diabetes Association. Position Statement: Foot care in patients with diabetes mellitus. *Diabetes Care.* 1998;21(Suppl 1):554–5.

37. Armstrong DG, Lavery LA, Harkless LB, op. cit.

38. Mayfield JA, Reiber GE, Sanders LJ, Janisse D, Pogach LM. Preventive foot care in people with diabetes. *Diabetes Care.* 1998;21(12):2161–77.

39. Litzelman DK, Marriot DJ, Vinicor F, op. cit.

40. American Diabetes Association. Consensus Development Conference on Diabetic Foot Wound Care (Consensus Statement). *Diabetes Care.* 1999;22(8):1354–60.

41. American Diabetes Association. Clinical Practice Recommendations: Preventive foot care in people with diabetes. *Diabetes Care.* 2000;23(Suppl 1) 1: S55–6.

42. National Diabetes Education Program. *Feet Can Last a Lifetime: A Health Care Provider's Guide to Preventing Diabetes Foot Problems, 2000,* rev. 2001. Accessed 4/06/07 at http://ndep.nih.gov/diabetes/pubs/Feet_Kit_Eng.pdf.

43. National Institute of Diabetes and Digestive and Kidney Diseases. *National Diabetes Statistics.* NIH Publication No. 02-3892, revised 2002. Accessed 4/06/07 at: http://diabetes.niddk.nih.gov/dm/pubs/statistics/#7.

44 Thomann KH, Marks ES, Adamczyk DT. *Primary Eyecare in Systemic Disease,* 2nd ed. New York: McGraw-Hill; 2001, p. 189–204.

45. Diabetes Control and Complications Trial Research Group, op. cit.

46. Chew EY, Klein ML, Murphy RP, Remaley NA, Ferris FL III, Early Treatment Diabetic Retinopathy Study Research Group: Effects of aspirin on preretinal hemorrhage in patients with diabetes mellitus. ETDRS Report Number 20. *Arch Ophthalmol* 113: 52–55, 1995.

47. Early Treatment Diabetic Retinopathy Study Research Group: Effects of aspirin treatment on diabetic retinopathy. ETDRS Report Number 8. *Ophthalmology* 98: 757–765, 1991.

48. Flynn HW Jr, Chew EY, Simons BD, Barton FB, Remaley NA, Ferris FL III. Pars plana vitrectomy in the Early Treatment Diabetic Retinopathy Study. ETDRS Report Number 17. The Early Treatment Diabetic Retinopathy Study Research Group. *Ophthalmology* 1992:99(9):1351–1357.

49. Loe H. Periodontal disease. The sixth complication of diabetes mellitus. *Diabetes Care* 1993;16:329–34.

50. U.S. Department of Health and Human Services. *Oral Health in America: A Report of the Surgeon General.* Rockville, MD: U.S. Department of Health and Human Services, National Institutes of Health, National Institute of Dental and Craniofacial Research, 2000.

51. Mealey BL, Oates TW. Diabetes Mellitus and Periodontal Diseases. *J Periodontol* 2006;77:1289–1303.

52. Tsai C, Hayes C, Taylor GW. Glycemic control of type 2 diabetes and severe periodontal disase in the U.S. adult population. *Community Dent Oral Epidemiol* 2002; 30:182–92.

53. Southerland JH, Taylor GW, Offenbacher S. Diabetes and periodontal infection: Making the connection. *Clinical Diabetes* 2005; 23(4):171–178.

54. Mealey, op. cit.

55. U.S. DHHS, 2000, op. cit.

56. Taylor GW. Bidirectional interrelationships between diabetes and periodontal diseases: An epidemiologic perspective. *Ann Periodontol* 2001;6(1):99–112.

57. Grossi SG, Genco RJ. Periodontal disease and diabetes mellitus: Two-way relationship. *Ann Periodontol* 1998;3(1):51–61.

58. Grossi SG, Skrepcinski FB, DeCaro T, Robertson DC, Ho AW, Dunford RG. Treatment of periodontal disease in diabetics reduces glycated hemoglobin. *J Periodontol* 1997;68 (8):713–9.

59. Taylor GW, Burt BA, Becker MP, Genco RJ, Shlossman M, Knowler WC, Pettitt DJ. Severe periodontitis and risk for poor glycemic control in patients with non-insulin-dependent diabetes mellitus. *J Periodontol* 1996;67(10 Suppl):1085–93.

60. Iacopino AM. Periodontitis and diabetes interrelationships: Role of inflammation. *Ann Periodontol* 2001;6(1):125–37.

61. Donahue RP, Wu T. Insulin resistance and periodontal disease: An epidemiologic overview of research needs and future directions. *Ann Periodontol* 2001;6(1):119–24.

62. Ernst FR, Grizzle AJ. Drug-related morbidity and mortality: Updating the cost of illness model. *J Am Pharm Assoc* 2001;41:192–9.

63. Johnson JA, Bootman JL. Drug-related morbidity and mortality. A cost-of-illness model. *Arch Intern Med* 1995;155(18):1949–56.

64. Bootman JL. The $76 billion wake-up call. *J Am Pharm Assoc (Wash)* 1996 Jan;NS36(1):27–8.

65. Saydah SH, Fradkin J, Cowie CC. Poor control of risk factors for vascular disease among adults with previously diagnosed diabetes. *JAMA* 2004;291(3):335–342.

66. Galt KA. Cost avoidance, acceptance, and outcomes associated with a pharmacotherapy consult clinic in a Veterans Affairs Medical Center. *Pharmacotherapy* 1998;8(5):1103–11.

67. Bluml BM, McKenney JM, Cziraky MJ. Pharmaceutical care services and results in project ImPACT: Hyperlipidemia. *J Am Pharm Assoc*, 2000;40(2):157–65.

68. Tsuyuki RT, Johnson JA, Teo KK, Simpson SH, Ackman ML, Biggs RS, Cave A, Chang WC, Dzavik V, Farris KB, et al. A randomized trial of the effect of community pharmacist intervention on cholesterol risk management: The Study of Cardiovascular Risk Intervention by Pharmacists (SCRIP). *Arch Intern Med* 2002;162(10):1149–55.

69. Yeh G, Eisenberg D, Davis R, Phillips R, Use of complementary and alternative medicine among persons with diabetes mellitus: Results of a national survey. *American Journal of Public Health*, 2002: 92:1648-1652.

70. Borgsdorf LR, Miano JS, Knapp KK. Pharmacist-managed medication review in a managed care system. *Am J Hosp Pharm* 1994;51:772–7.

71. Hitchcock AM, Lousberg TR, Merenich J. The impact of clinical pharmacy management on cardiovascular risk reduction in patients with established heart disease in a group model health maintenance organization. *Pharmacotherapy* 2000;20:360–1, abstract 135.

72. Johnson JA, Bootman JL, op. cit.

73. Bluml BM, McKenney JM, Cziraky MJ, op. cit.

74. American Diabetes Association. Clinical practice recommendations. *Diabetes Care* 2006;29(Suppl 1):S12. http://care.diabetesjournals.org/content/vol29/suppl_1/.

75. American Diabetes Association. Clinical practice recommendations. *Diabetes Care* 2006;29(Suppl 1) http://care.diabetesjournals.org/content/vol29/suppl_1/.

76. American Diabetes Association. Clinical
    practice recommendations. *Diabetes
    Care* 2006;29(Suppl 1) http://care.
    diabetesjournals.org/content/vol29/
    suppl_1/.

77. Ibid.

78. Ibid.

79. Centers for Medicare & Medicaid
    Services. *General Program Description*.
    Accessed 4/06/07 at: http://www.cms.
    hhs.gov/clia/01_overview.asp.